Celebrity Trainer
Christianne Wolff

The Body Rescue Plan

bodyresc♥e

ISBN 978-1-910125-29-8

With thanks to...

The Cooks: Mum and Marie-Francoise for helping me cook all the recipes for the photo shoot.

The Photographers: Nikki Sheffield (lifestyle), Paul Magee (Food), Andreas Le-sauvage (Fitness and lifestyle)

CD recording and composing: Simon Lague

The Book Designer: Gary Alake Riley, Tabloid Tomato Design

Acknowledgements

My husband Robbie, who always believes in me and thinks I can and will do anything.

My most beautiful bundle of joy, Angelique Amberley, who is my life and my love and I adore you.

My wonderful parents who gave me the most amazing upbringing and have inspired me in every way imaginable. From the organic food that bursts through their house, to their amazing vegetable patches and home grown fruits. Both their endless creativity and inspiration, youthfulness and fun. To their dedication to their own spiritual beliefs, and their passion for helping others less fortunate than them. They gave me space so I could breathe, create and love and I thank you, Mum and Dad, so much for that, you are pure love. x

My amazing brothers and sisters who are..

Michele, for your utter inspiration on anything health-related, you have inspired me all my life.

Tim, Paul, Suzie, Andrew and Marie-Francoise for always being there for me and being incredible.

To my cousin Nicola, who is always supportive and makes me laugh more than anyone.

To Liz Green, my amazing spiritual mentor and lover of life, thank you for your humble teachings.

And to all my clients past and present, who have given me hours of fun, intellect, inspiration, and put food on my table.

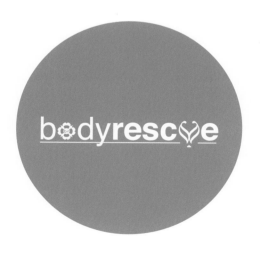

Christianne and The Body Rescue Plan in the Press...

"After 12 weeks I'd lost over 2 stone and gone from a size 16 to a 12 (UK). I'm the fittest and healthiest I've ever been and I'm determined to stay that way"

Mernie Gilmore
Womans editor, The Daily Express

"The Body Rescue plan is so comprehensively structured, that this has made it so much easier to self-motivate. The diet and exercise has meant I toned my arms and abs within weeks, after years of half-hearted trying. I particularly like the integration of yoga and mindfulness into the plan, which I think has been key to making it work for me"

Jessica Elgot
Assitant Editor, Huffington Post

"I am suitably inspired by Christianne Wolff, whose Body Rescue Plan book is now published"

The Daily Telegraph

"Get fit, healthy and lose weight with The Body Rescue Plan which has been created by award-winning celebrity trainer, Christianne Wolff. Using spiritual and relaxation practices, combined with fitness routines, healthy diet plans and the mindset to heal old patterns, the plan has helped people lose weight and gain confidence in just 12 weeks."

Woman and home magazine

"Party dress workout, don't panic! There's still time to look fabulous for your Christmas party. We asked personal trainer Christianne Wolff for her best moves! (from The Body Rescue Plan)"

OK magazine

"Tone your stomach in two weeks with Christianne Wolff, in this exercises from The Body Rescue Plan."

Reveal Magazine

"Hone your physique with the total body workout devised by celebrity trainer Christianne Wolff."

Body Fit magazine

"Christianne Wolff recommends top ways to make sure your fitness and energy levels rise."

Hello magazine

"The Body Rescue Plan Made Me The Slimmest I've Been Since I was 18".

HuffPost

"The Body Rescue Plan has over 50 healthy recipes and teaches how you can lose 2.5 stone in 12 weeks through fitness, yoga and detox."

Workout magazine

"Christianne Wolff is the author of The Body Rescue, slimming, mindset and fitness plan and is THE perfect weight loss plan."

Ultra Fit magazine

"Christianne's plan gives you mood boosting energy."

Healthy magazine

"Lose up to 10 pounds in the first 2 weeks and feel fantastic with Christianne Body Rescue Plan, this plan is really simple and you will not go hungry."

Express online

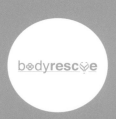

"Kiss your flab goodbye, with Christianne's mood lifting workout"

Cosmopolitan

"Face facts its hard to get motivated when exercising at home, but fret not Christianne has ways for you to tone up at home"

**Celebs on Sunday
(Daily Mirror)**

"Christianne Wolff puts a glittering list of high profile clients through their paces, in a bid to keep them lean and lovely"

Mens Fitness

"Christianne reveals the golden rules, her celebrity clients have to adhere to and offers crucial advice"

Celebrity homes

"Want a trainer but can't afford to stump up the cash? Then go to celebrity trainer Christianne Wolff "

Zest

"Get a behind like Pippa Middleton, with celebrity trainer Christianne Wolff"

Daily Mirror

"I went to The Chilterns 'Body Rescue' studio of Christianne Wolff, personal trainer to actors and high profile businessmen/women- Christianne has taught me to shake up my fitness regime and rethink what I am trying to achieve."

FT Times

"Celebrity personal trainer Christianne Wolff has created an at-home workout to enhance your six pack"

The Daily Express

" Try these exercises to help improve your posture -from Christianne Wolff, they are excellent for strengthening the core-stability muscles that wrap around our middle and help to support the lumbar spine"

The Guardian

"Is she a personal trainer or an angel? Christianne, you are a bonafide fitness genius."

Sweaty Betty

"If she can get me to exercise then she really can get anyone to!"

**Martha Lane Fox
Lastminute.com**

"Health on my shelf with Celebrity trainer, healer and motivational speaker Christianne Wolff"

Womans Weekly

"Christianne runs chilterns most prestigious personal training gym"

Eve magazine

"Christianne has worked with Bond movie stars and championship motorcyclists. She wears those annoying little crop tops and possesses an extraordinarily pert bottom, Christianne was a different prospect entirely, she makes getting fit more fun."

**Mimi Spencer
Evening Standard**

Foreword

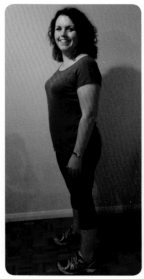
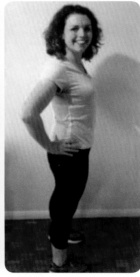

Do you want to lose weight? Have you tried lots of diets before? Do you feel stuck with bad eating habits and not sure how to change them? Are you fed up feeling unhappy with the way you look?

I'd certainly felt all these things at one time or another before I started the Body Rescue plan.
I had two stone to lose but couldn't shift it. I knew I wasn't eating a particularly healthy diet but I couldn't motivate myself to change it.

Then Christianne stepped in and told me if I followed her programme I could lose that weight in just 12 weeks. I'll admit I was intrigued - but I still didn't think I'd be able to do it.

When I read the first two weeks of the diet plan my fears were confirmed. No sugar? No alcohol? No caffeine? I thought there was no way I'd be able to give them up.

But with summer looming I was determined to do something and with Christianne's encouragement I started the programme.

I'm not going to lie. The first week was tough. But by the end of the week the headaches had lifted and I started to feel better. And a few days after that I felt great.

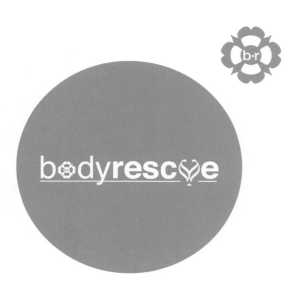

I started sleeping well. Whereas before it had often taken me a long time to fall asleep, I was suddenly out like a light the moment my head hit the pillow. When I woke up in the morning I didn't feel tired and as the weeks went by my energy levels soared.

And then there was the weight loss. In the first two weeks alone I lost 8lb and after that it just kept coming off. Within a fortnight my eating habits had changed completely. Despite being on a "diet", I didn't feel hungry. By cutting out unnecessary sugar, I stopped craving it. I stopped grazing on food throughout the day and instead focused on eating healthy, nutritious meals.

I followed Christianne's advice about exercise, mixing cardio workouts with resistance exercises. I started doing yoga and pilates.

Despite initially being a bit sceptical about the more alternative elements such as visualisation and positive thinking I did them anyway. And do you know what? They worked. Within a few weeks I felt different. Happier, calmer and confident I was going to succeed.

If diets in the past have left you feeling miserable or you think you can't achieve your goal, then this could be the plan for you. The whole ethos behind Body Rescue is learning to feel good about yourself. The plan is full of brilliant exercises to help boost self-esteem and confidence while encouraging you to be kinder to yourself rather than critical.

As the weeks go on you'll find the way you look at yourself has changed.

After 12 weeks I'd lost over 2 stone and gone from a size 16 to a 12 (UK). I'm the fittest and healthiest I've ever been and I'm determined to stay that way.

Not only has the Body Rescue Plan changed the way I eat, it's changed the way I look, feel and think about myself. It's changed my life and I honestly believe it can change yours too.

Mernie Gilmore
Women's editor, Daily Express

About the author

Christianne Wolff is an award-winning celebrity trainer, yoga and Pilates instructor, writer and healer. She is internationally recognised as one of the leading experts in fitness and weight loss, and is particularly passionate about combining spiritual and relaxation practices with the fitness routine, using mindset to heal old patterns, in her unique Body Rescue Plan.

Christianne writes several columns for the national press and has appeared in over one hundred national magazines over the last seventeen years. She has trained many celebrities and hundreds of clients over the last two decades.

Christianne owns The Body Rescue Fitness and Well-being centres with her husband Robbie, and they run Luxury Detox and Fitness holidays around the world.

For more information on Christianne, go to www.thebodyrescueplan.com

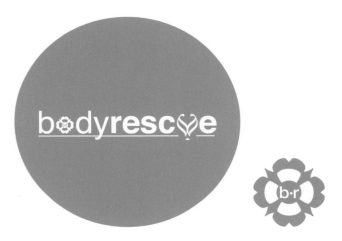

Disclaimer: Before starting this programme you may wish to seek medical advice from a doctor and get permission to start The Body Rescue Plan. The advice and instruction in The Body Rescue Plan does not replace any medical procedure and if the programme is not performed correctly could cause injury, as with any plan. Christianne Wolff disclaims any liability or loss.

First published in Great Britain in 2014. Text copyright © 2014 Christianne Wolff

Christianne Wolff is hereby identified as the author of this work in accordance with the copyright, designs and patents Act 1988.

Printed and bound in the UK

First Published 2014

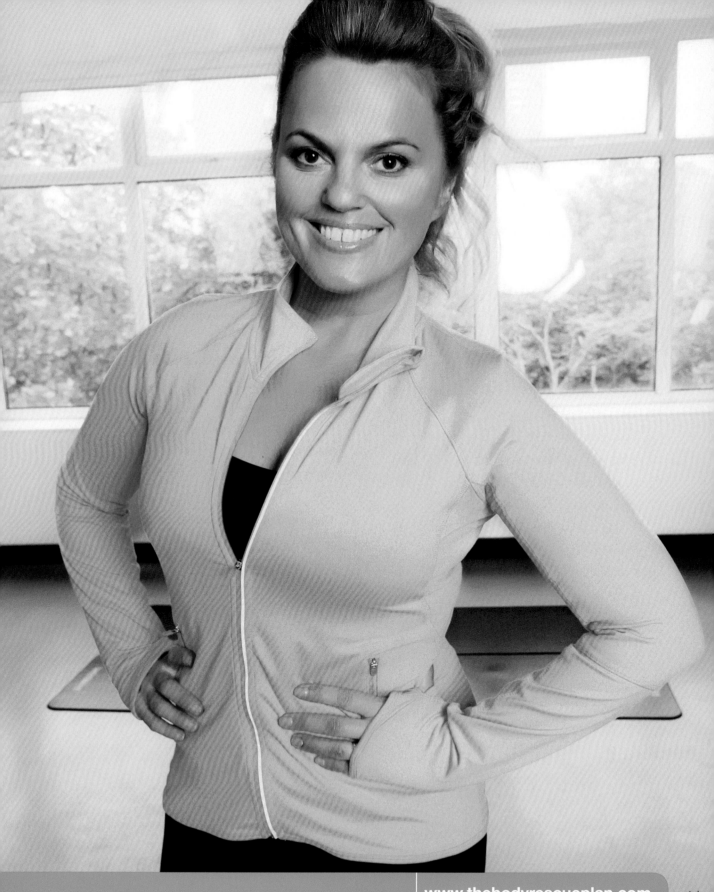

Contents

Chapter 1 - Introduction   **16**

My story

Chapter 2 - The 11 Golden Rules   **22**

01: Why Body rescue?   24

02: Questions and Answers   26

03: Testimonials   28

Chapter 3 - Mindset

01: Goals   45

02: Desire statements   48

03: Language and willpower   49

04: Trigger points   50

05: Avoiding pain versus confronting fear   53

06: Unhealthy priorities   55

07: Limiting beliefs   56

08: Guided meditations with visualisations   60

09: The Body Rescue Plan Meditations are..   62

10: Vision boarding   64

11: Gratitude   66

Chapter 4- Why Detox?   **69**

01: How to detox   70

02: Wheat and gluten   71

03: Dairy   72

04: Alcohol   72

05: Sugar   72

06: Other reasons to detox   73

07: Bath products   74

08: Other products   75

09: Foods that help a detox   75

10: Supplements and foods that can
    help you in a detoxification   79

11: Foods to avoid to cut belly fat   79

12: Sleep   80

13: Water   81

Chapter 5 - The Detox programme   **83**

Chapter 6 - The Body Rescue Diet Plan   **89**

01: Get organised   90

02: Creating associations   90

03: A note about breakfast   91

04: Weeks 1-12 eating plan   92

05: Maintenance   93

Chapter 7- Recipes and shopping list   **95**

01: Breakfast recipes 1   96

02: Smoothies & Juices   97

03: Breakfast recipes 2   99

04: Lunch and Supper recipes   100

05: Yummy snacks and puddings   108

06: Body Rescue Diet Plan   113

07: 7 day Body Rescue Diet Plan recipes   118

08: Shopping list   126

Chapter 8 -The Body Rescue Exercise Plan

01: Why exercise?   131

02: The best way to burn fat   133

03: The quickest workout   135

04: Choosing exercises   136

05: Warm-up exercises   136

06: Abdominal workout 1   138

07: Explanation of moves   139

08: Cardiovascular training   141

09: Interval training 1   142

10: Explanation of moves   143

11: Resistance workout 1   144

12: Explanation of moves   145

13: Abdominal workout 2   146

14: Explanation of moves   147

15: Interval training 2   148

16: Explanation of moves   149

17: Resistance workout 2   150

18: Explanation of moves   151

19: Stretch   152

20: Exercise programme   153

Chapter 9 - Yoga and meditation   **159**

01: Why Yoga?   160

02: Free Meditation CD download   162

03: The Body Rescue Yoga Chart   164

04: Explanation of the Yoga postures   166

Chapter 10
-Your Body Rescue Weekly Plan   **171**

Charts Weeks 1-13   174-199

Celebrity Trainer
Christianne Wolff
The Body Rescue Plan

Dedication

I dedicate this book in loving memory to my best friend Rebecca, you were always an amazing source of inspiration to me, and there is not a day that goes by where I don't think about you. Look at me, I wrote a book :)

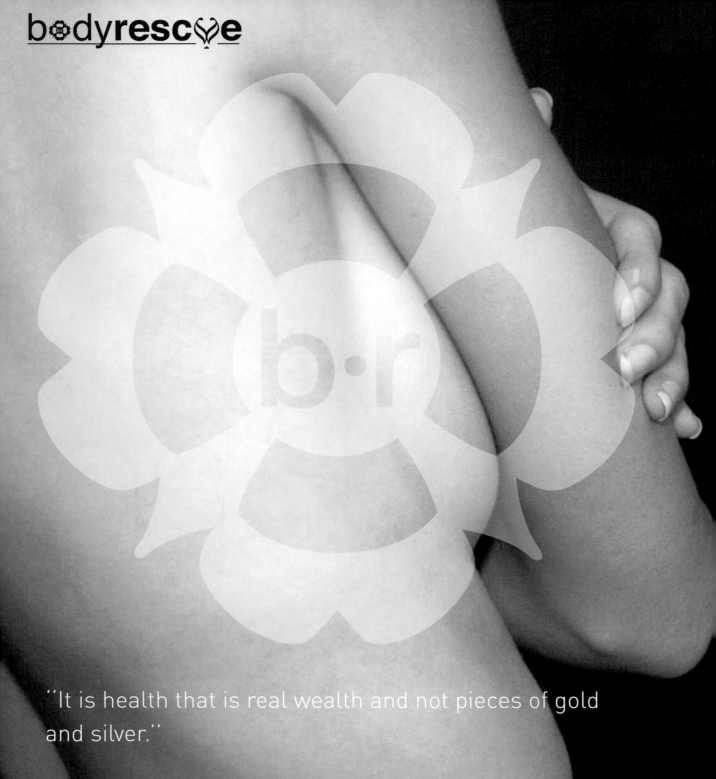

bodyrescue

"It is health that is real wealth and not pieces of gold and silver."

Mahatma Ghandi

Chapter 1

Introduction

My story

My story

Growing up

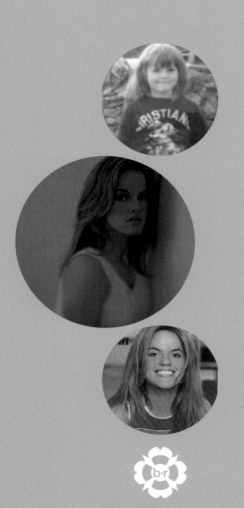

I had a wonderful, active childhood, climbing trees, cycling and dancing- but I was also often ill with bladder and kidney infections from the age of 4 and seemed to be continually on antibiotics. This had a terrible impact on my digestion and concentration levels as I got older. By my teens the only thing I could focus on at school was art and sports. I found it so hard to concentrate in other lessons that I would often get sent out of class. Needless to say my academic performance was very neglected and this lead to bouts of depression, suspension and expulsion from my school. By the age of 16 I felt I lived in a constant fog so I decided I had to do something about it. I started researching the effects of antibiotics and toxins on the body and this lead on to my love affair with health, nutrition and fitness. I also realised that the type of sport I was doing was just anaerobic so I then bought 3 fitness videos that I practiced from religiously every week. They were Jerry Halls yoga video, Jane Fondas aerobics video and Calanetics! I put myself on a sugar, dairy and yeast free diet and I started to see some quite miraculous results. Newfound concentration levels meant I was able to read a full book for the first time in my life and my energy levels soared. I went on to college and university to study a degree in 3D Design and it was the first time I really thrived. I was successful and I was fit.

I started teaching aerobics in the 1990s.
By then I had realised that my depressed feelings lifted when I exercised, particularly when I did cardiovascular training. My digestion was normal and the fog had disappeared. I could even eat some naughty foods from time to time without hyperactivity or restlessness. I had such a strong passion for fitness and health and helping people get well again that in 1997 I qualified and became a personal trainer.

As a trainer I soon noticed an exercise-based training programme wasn't enough for my clients.
To achieve their goals they needed emotional support, nutritional advice, deep stretching and to develop a real connection and love of themselves. So I went on to study further and became a teacher in yoga, meditation and pilates, life coaching, a reiki master and a published writer.

I then went on to be a magazine columnist for Mens Fitness and presented on TV shows on Sky TV and ITV for fitness and well being.

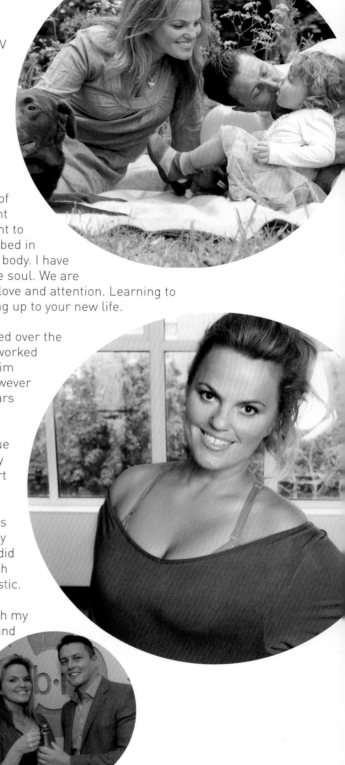

Now I own the Body Rescue Fitness and Wellbeing centres with my husband Robbie Wood, a former professional footballer who is now a trainer and physiotherapist. I have trained hundreds of people over the last 17 years, from celebrities on film sets, pop stars preparing for their tours, athletes training for their seasons,
to housewives and people just like you. The majority of my clients come to me not only wanting to lose weight but to feel more alive. They are stuck in a rut and want to have a better quality of life. They want to jump out of bed in the morning, look in the mirror and be proud of their body. I have always believed in training the mind, the body and the soul. We are complicated creatures and need to be nurtured with love and attention. Learning to embrace that love will be the start of you really waking up to your new life.

I have written this book using everything I have learned over the last 20 years, what I have seen that has and has not worked for my clients and also myself. I am not a naturally slim person, I have a naturally curvy, hourglass figure. However I have had a flat stomach and toned body over the years because I have worked for it.

In 2010 I gave birth to my beautiful daughter Angelique Amberley. I trained and taught classes throughout my pregnancy and even walked the Ivinghoe Beacon (part of the Ridgeway walk) when I was 10 days overdue in the hope she would come out. In the end it took another five days beyond that, to this day she still likes to keep me waiting! I lost weight fairly quickly after my pregnancy and got back into training straight away. I did pilates and my body rescue plan to flatten my stomach and after a year I trained for a triathlon and felt fantastic.

Soon after my triathlon I found out I was pregnant with my second child. My husband and I were over the moon and began preparing our new life for our larger family. At the time I was teaching a variety of yoga, pilates and zumba classes a week but during one of the zumba classes I realised something was wrong. I went to hospital with Robbie and a few days later I was given the awful news I had miscarried. Going through the miscarriage was horrendous. Even though it was early on in the pregnancy I already felt connected to my baby, I felt she was a girl and had dark hair. I could see her and now she was gone. It felt as if the doctors just expected me to pick up and carry on as if nothing had happened whereas inside I was devastated.

To make things worse, this had all happened while I was exercising... The exercise I loved, that brought me out of depression, gave me energy and a zest for life was suddenly associated with the worst feeling in the world and a loss I can't describe. Of course the zumba class did not contribute to the miscarriage in any way but my subconscious wouldn't let it go and I stopped all my classes except yoga and within a year I put on 1st 7lb. Then I developed a stomach condition, which made my stomach bloat so badly I couldn't even drive on some occasions as it was like being 9 months pregnant, and this lead to another 14 pound weight gain. I was 2.5 stone over weight and felt awful. The crunch time came when a well known celebrity I knew asked me if my sister was my daughter!-I was looking old and fat and I knew I had to do something about it.

I needed to work on my mindset techniques to break this cycle. I tried to get back into my old routine of eating healthy and exercising but it would only last for week or so before I felt negative again.

I had taught meditation for years but decided to devise a series of meditation techniques for myself to really grasp what I was going through. I wanted to feel positive about exercise again, to get rid of the guilt and shame about what had happened, to calm me down and boost my willpower. Within 12 weeks of starting this my weight was down by 2.5 stone (35 pounds), my skin was young and clear, my eyes were bright and my flat abs were back. My mind was strong again and soon I was training every day and loving it again. I knew my techniques worked and I began trying them on my clients, offering them my CDs or treating them in person with healing which had incredible results.

Most weight loss books barely touch on working with your emotions and your mindset, or balancing your hormones or embracing love. But most people with weight issues have mind issues too, often linked to self esteem and self worth. I think any weight loss programme has to be about feeling good, about your health, your life and most importantly, yourself. The looking good bit is a by-product of that. This is why I have written The Body Rescue slimming, mindset and fitness plan. This is years of research, studying and trialling through my clients to what I have found to be the perfect weight loss plan.

What I can promise you is that if you follow my plan you will find:
- A simple diet that is easy and sustainable.
- Exercise routines that are fun and progress as you improve.
- That your mind is happy so you want more.
- That you are calm and controlled and not doing this for a quick fix.
- And that the food is delicious in texture, taste, colour and smells.

The results on this programme will astonish you. You will lose up to 10lb in the first two weeks and then 1lb to 3lb a week thereafter until you reach my maintenance programme. Not only that, but your body and your mind will improve in every way so that you feel like a new person. A person in control, who has beauty, energy, health and love. All you have to look forward to is a fitter, happier, more gorgeous version of you!

Enjoy
Christianne xxx

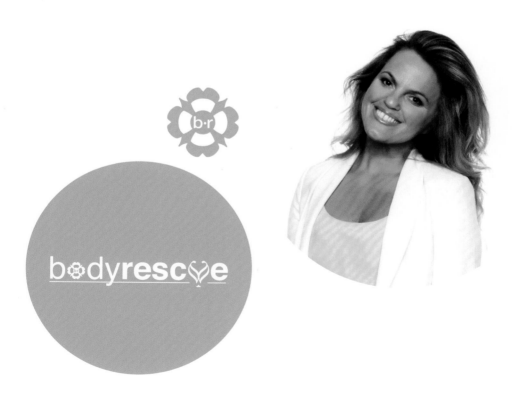

"Clarity is a beautiful thing!
Even if you had to go through a storm to get there."
Christianne Wolff

Chapter 2
The Body Rescue Plan

01: The 11 Golden Rules of The Body Rescue Plan

02: Why Body Rescue?

03: Questions & answers

04: Testimonials

01: The 11 Golden Rules of The Body Rescue Plan.

There are 11 main components to my programme.
Follow them and you will be on your way to the body of your dreams, have loads of energy and feel amazing.

1 Do my detox for 2 weeks
The first two weeks of the plan helps to cleanse the body and get rid of toxins.

2 Do my 10 week eating plan
Full of delicious foods that will fill you up and make you feel full of energy and youth.

3 Do my mindset programme
To set goals and reprogramme your brain. It will boost your willpower, banish addictions to sugar and caffeine and establish a whole range of new good eating habits.

4 Get at least seven hours sleep a night
There is a lot of research which has shown a link between lack of sleep and weight gain, so make an effort to get as much shut-eye as possible. If you have always struggled to nod off you will find it much easier when you given up caffeine.

5 Drink plenty of water
Being hydrated is essential for good health, weight loss and drinking water curbs your appetite.

6 Cut out caffeine

Caffeine is a diuretic so it can affect your weight loss as you are dehydrated. It can also affect your insulin levels which means you crave carbs after the initial stimulation has worn off.

7 Cut out sugar

Sugar plays havoc with your blood sugar levels which makes you eat. The more you have the more you want it. Giving up sugar is like giving up a drug, once its out of your system you no longer crave it.

8 Plan your mindset, exercise and meals

Making a plan for the week about what you will eat and when you will exercise has been proven to make or break a fitness and diet programme. There will always be an excuse if you are tired or get a better offer but if you firmly plan out your week then you will achieve your results.

9 Do resistance/interval training work

Many people do cardiovascular training such as running, cycling or aerobics thinking it's the only way to burn fat and lose weight. However resistance training and interval training are essential for weight loss too, so are an integral part of my programme.

10 Find exercise you enjoy

Making your exercise programme fun will help you sustain in the long term. There are so many things you can do from out door swimming, to mountain biking.

11 Do yoga, relax and focus on you

For many reasons stress makes you fat! Stress affects the levels of cortisol (the stress hormone) in your body. This can lead to cravings and eating when you're not hungry. Research also suggests that cortisol can make you hold on to fat around your middle.

Taking up meditation or yoga makes you take time out to breathe, stretch and relax, perfect to keep stress levels down and allow yourself to focus on you.

02: Why Body Rescue?

The Body Rescue plan is a 12 week plan.
You Get ...

- A 2 week detox programme
- Mindset programming with 6 meditations on a download from www.thebodyrescueplan.com for life
- A 10 week diet programme
- Over 50 recipes
- A weeks menu plan with a shopping list
- A 12 week exercise programme with progressive exercises and photos
- A yoga programme with photos
- A 12 week full chart plan

What body rescue is NOT..

- A starvation and binge diet.. instead you will learn manageable ways to deal with addictions to foods, and balancing moods.

- A low fat diet..instead you will learn that fat is really important for your nutritional health and not all fats are the same.

- A low calorie diet.. instead you are able to eat freely many wonderful delicious foods. Low calorie diets don't work and leave your body holding onto fat!

- A non carb diet..you can eat as much fruit as you like and still eat your favourite carb meals.

- A diet where you can never eat certain foods ever again..instead once you are on the maintenance programme you are able to eat what you like on one day a week.

- An advocate for diet foods.. instead you will re-fuel your body with the foods and nutrition it so badly craves.

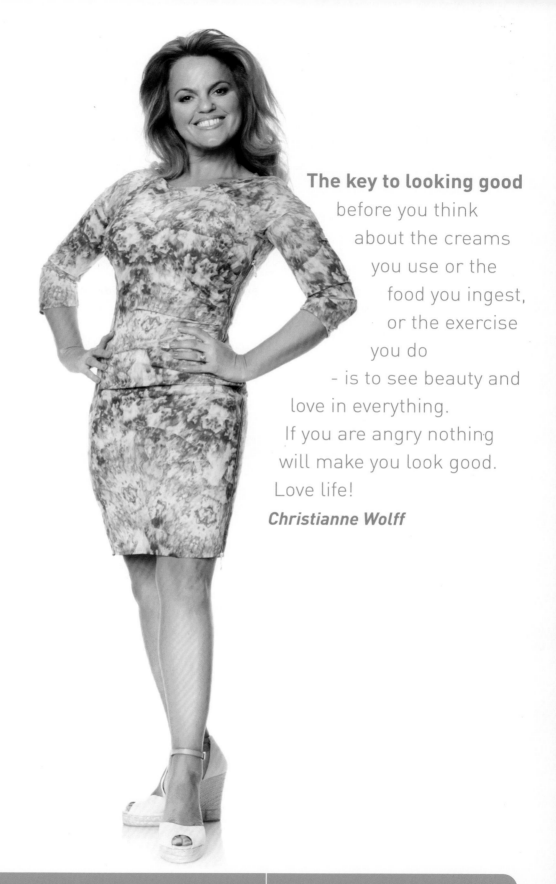

The key to looking good before you think about the creams you use or the food you ingest, or the exercise you do - is to see beauty and love in everything. If you are angry nothing will make you look good. Love life!

Christianne Wolff

03: Questions & answers

Isn't Fruit full of sugar?
The sugar in fruit is not refined sugar, fruit is full of vitamins and fibre and the sugar found in fruit does not have the same effect on the body as refined sugar. I suggest eating more vegetables than fruit as a way to not go over board with fruit consumption.

Why can you eat nuts and seeds, I thought they were really fattening?
Nuts and seeds are full of the good fats, and we need these in our diets to help with absorbing certain vitamins, these are essential to our health. Only have 1 fist full a day.

Can I do the Body Rescue Plan if I am breastfeeding or pregnant?
No. The Body Rescue plan is a weight loss and detox programme that is not suitable if you are pregnant or breastfeeding.

Can I have milk?
No, there is no cows milk on the whole 12 week plan, you may have milk in the maintenance plan on 1 day a week. However you are allowed oat, rice or almond week after the detox.

I have high blood pressure/I am not in good health, is this suited to me?
If you have any doubts about your fitness and health please contact the Doctors prior to doing The Body Rescue Plan to check you are fit and healthy enough.

Will I cope giving up caffeine and sugar- where will I get my energy from?
You will have more energy than you have ever had. Once the toxins are out of your system (3-5 days) you will feel amazing and will start resourcing into your natural energies.

Can I really have as much fruit as I want?
Yes, provided you have more vegetables/salad than fruit.

Are all herbal teas ok?
Most are fine, just make sure they do not have caffeine in- green tea does have caffeine in so should be avoided for 12 weeks.

What do I do if I get ill or injured?
As this is a 12 week programme you may get a cold, flu or sickness bug during this time period. If you feel well enough, keep doing the abdominal programme and perhaps go for a walk, but rest as much as possible. No matter what your illness is you can still stick with the mindset programme, using it to help you get better. To help prevent an injury you must always warm up and cool down in any workout and stretch at the end. Tension and stress often relates to illness and injury, and as this programme is all about releasing that from your body, you should find you are a lot more healthy as a result.

04: Testimonials

Find out from my clients how the Body Rescue Plan changed their lives.

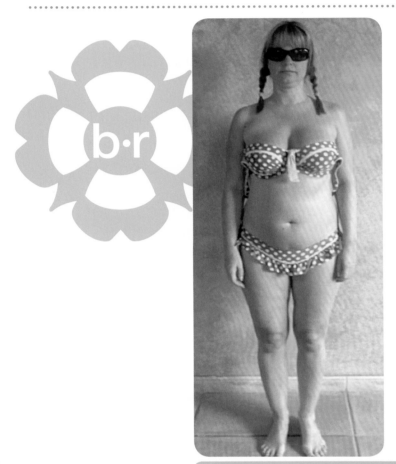

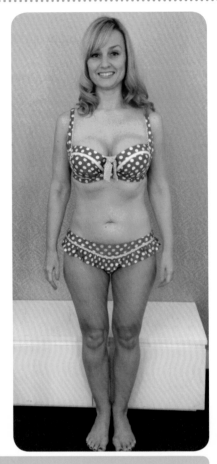

Catherine after 12 weeks!

"I lost 2.5stone in 12 weeks on The Body Rescue Plan and went from a size 16 to a size 10.

After enduring decades of issues with fluctuating weight, body image & nutrition I have finally found the perfect lifelong plan for me.

Over the years I have gone from size 6 to size 16. This hadn't been a steady, upwards progression but a cycle of going up rapidly and then down just as quickly and back again. I have been, like so many, a 'yo-yo' dieter. I have, indeed, tried many diets and they have worked well in so much as I lost weight doing them, however, once I reached the weight or size I wanted I found it hard to maintain. They served their purpose to reach a short term goal for a special event but, for me, they weren't ever going to be the long term solution I needed.

I had major issues with food. At times I would survive on one banana a day and other times I would binge, sometimes eating a whole cheesecake or fast food at breakfast time and take aways night after night. I even ordered twice as much so I could have the same binge the next day

Catherine went from a size 16 to a size 10 on The Body Rescue Plan.

for breakfast! Imagine my poor arteries!

Previous diets involved counting calories, tiny portions, flavourless foods and, in the main, a general feeling of deprivation. Even when I found systems which worked better for me I didn't feel 'well'. I often felt shaky and I certainly wasn't in shape as I never fully committed to exercise. I had become a master of disguise. No one could ever really appreciate just how out of shape or large I had become as I used every trick in the book to conceal it from the world. I would double up on support garments, wear maximum coverage clothing and the highest heels I could find in order to look slimmer. I also deprived myself of many social events as I was too depressed about how I felt I looked. It's been a struggle to find any photos of me at my most unhealthy due to the fact I would ask friends to delete them. This year I turned 42. It dawned on my that if I continued this way not only would I carry on being enslaved by food but my health was beginning to suffer and I could be headed towards an early grave. I was considering seeking professional help when I was introduced to Christianne. Christianne was very honest and told me she needed 100% commitment from me. I was ready to commit. I wanted to change for life, not just for a bikini or occasion. More than anything I wanted my health so I could be around for my children as long as possible. I was 25 when my father died due to heart disease. There's so much he's missed out on and so much we've missed by not having him here. The greatest tribute to his memory I can offer is to be well so I can see his grandchildren, my children, through all of their different life stages and maybe even, one day, become the

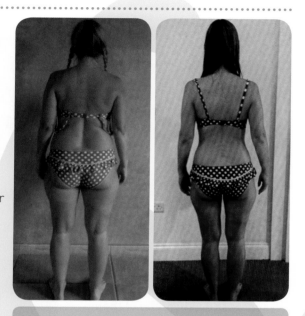

Catherine after 10 weeks!

healthy grandparent he didn't get the chance to be.

The new lease of life I have been given through using the Body Rescue Plan is beyond anything I can put into words.

The food tastes so much better now I've cut out sugar, I enjoy preparing and eating meals with my adult children and Christianne's recipes are absolutely delicious!! I make the time for my exercise and always feel better for doing it. I can finally see some tone and definition in my body. Even when I was a size 6 I wasn't toned, just malnourished!

I have recommended this plan to all of my friends. Many have committed and are achieving great results, too. If you're willing to commit you have so much more than weight loss to gain. This will always be the year I changed my life forever and I can't thank Christianne enough."

**Catherine Huntley
TV presenter**

04: Testimonials

Find out from my clients how the Body Rescue Plan changed their lives.

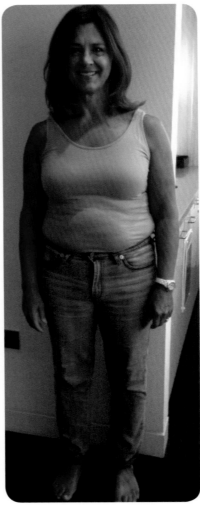

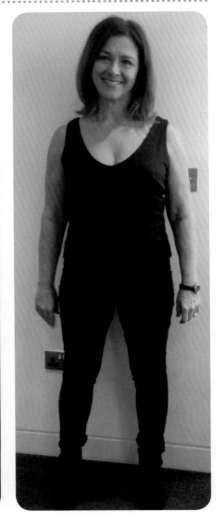

"I've tried many diets, and been successful with some of them - but only temporarily, and only to a certain point. I seem unable to keep going to my target weight, and I soon regain most of the lost weight. That's when I try the next diet!

Christianne's Body Rescue is different, and I am delighted to say - no, I'll shout it! - that after following Body Rescue for nine weeks I WEIGH LESS THAN I HAVE DONE FOR THE LAST 10 YEARS. It has helped me budge those last stubborn pounds. I've just reached the milestone of dropping by one stone and plan to lose seven more pounds to be my lightest ever for 20 years - since before the birth of my third child who is now a strapping 6 foot plus nineteen year old!

I think the reason Body Rescue works is that it's not just a diet. By integrating not just home exercises but yoga and, most importantly, mindfulness and visualisation, Christianne tackles the emotional reasons that so many of us carry more weight than we should. Acknowledging guilt and self sabotage, addressing and reducing the negative stress in our lives and recognising how low-self esteem can make sticking to a diet so much harder mean that Body Rescue is a complete programme, for body AND mind. And that is why it has worked for me!"

Kathy Tayler
TV presenter

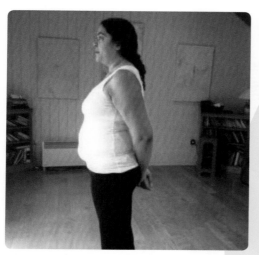
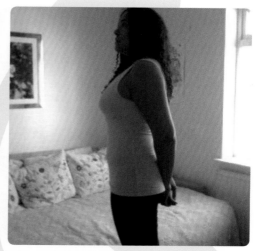

"I lost 2.5 stone with Christianne's Body Rescue detox, diet and exercise plan.
I loved the exercise plan, I loved the exercise plan, particularly the Pilates style exercise and some of the cardio and yes, definitely my body shape has changed. The exercises were easy to follow and I didn't need any fancy equipment.

The first week of detox was quite a challenge, the second week was a lot easier, and by the time I got to the maintenance plan I found it really easy and delicious.

I am far more conscious of what I put in my mouth and I am never hungry, I am generally satisfied after every meal and am no longer thinking about food all day long.

My energy levels were very low before I started this programme and now I feel worlds away from how I felt 3 months ago, and my complexion is the best it has ever been!!

My friends all tell me I look amazing, and I can't believe the difference.
If I can do it, anyone can do this, I have had a back injury to contend with and two young children."
Daniella Orchard
Owner of "The Little Orchard cafe"

Daniella lost over 2 stone on The Body Rescue Plan.

04: Testimonials

Find out from my clients how the Body Rescue Plan changed their lives.

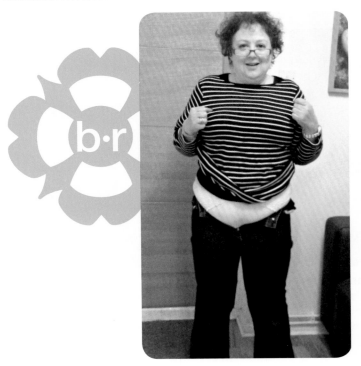

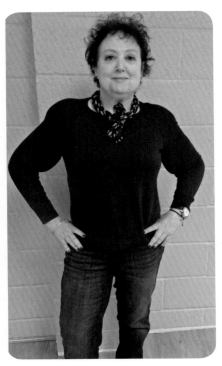

"I had spent a few days at a boot camp at the end of 2014 to help motivate me to improve my fitness and lose weight. I have been an asthma sufferer for about 6 years and had been diagnosed with Type 2 Diabetes for about a year. Whilst the boot camp was a great experience I knew I would need something that would educate me for the long term and keep me focussed on a daily basis.

I was looking for a plan; not a diet but a lifestyle regime when I came across the Body Rescue Plan.

I devoured the body rescue plan book in the first couple of weeks. For me the Food science was the most beneficial. As someone with a busy job that takes me away from home so much I had been a microwave addict. I never had any real interest in cooking and recipes, they always seemed so complicated and time consuming.

What surprised me and excited me about Christianne's food was how simple it was to make and how delicious the food.

I would make different versions of the same thing and cook on a Sunday for the whole week so if I came home from work late, all I would have to do is heat it up. For me planning my weekly meals is of the utmost importance. I particularly love the home made Muesli and the Lentil Curry.

The first two weeks were the hardest and giving up tea and coffee (I drunk about 6-7 mugs a day) was really hard but I got through it and can honestly say I don't miss it at all anymore. I found a love of hot water with lemon which I drink throughout the day. I no longer drink diet fizzy drinks and if I'm out for dinner I stick to mineral water. If I eat in a restaurant I tend to stick to Grilled fish and salad.

The section of the book on yoga and meditation was a new experience for me. I love the yoga and find I am bendier than I thought and love the stretching which relieves the tension as I spend a lot of time hunched over a steering wheel. The meditation I found a little more

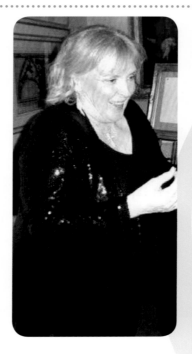

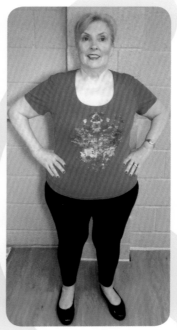

difficult as I am easily distracted and but I'm getting there.

My life has drastically changed in the past 12 weeks. Firstly I have lost 2 stone and whilst I still need to lose another 1 ½ stone I KNOW I am on the right track to lose it. I will remain on the plan until I lose the last bit.

Finally, the biggest change since being on the plan is that by blood sugar is now totally balanced and I am no longer Diabetic. After a recent blood test my Doctor looked at the results then looked at me (and my weight loss) and said *'I don't know what you're doing but whatever it is you're doing great and your blood sugar levels are perfect!'.*"

Cheryl Rose

"I have been on The Body Rescue Plan for 12 weeks. It is extremely simple to follow and I suffered no hungry feelings at all, which was marvellous, you can have some lovely recipes too. From week one the weight started to drop off.

In just 12 weeks, not only have I lost an amazing amount of weight, but my skin is so clear- I had terrible red flakey skin that completely cleared up after just 4-5 weeks. I also ran out of HRT whilst on the plan and noticed I had no side effects, which I never had before. I always had a strong reaction when I ran out- I decided to stay off HRT for a few weeks to see if it would continue and it did, after 12 weeks I still have no side effects. The transformation has been quite incredible and it's all down to The Body Rescue Plan! I have tried every diet out there to get the weight to come off and I can honestly say nothing has worked like The Body Rescue Plan - I feel 20 years younger!! In the 12 weeks, I have lost 2 stone 10 lbs and gone from a size 22 to a size 16/18!"

Stella Adams
Director at Exclusive Magazines

04: Testimonials

Find out from my clients how the Body Rescue Plan changed their lives.

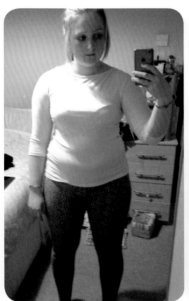 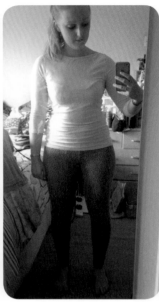 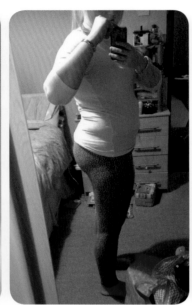 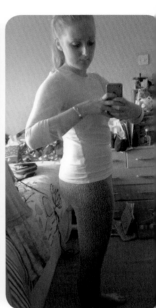

"The Body Rescue Plan has had a major impact on the foods I eat. It has introduced me to new foods that I would never have tried before and I have found some new favourites along the way!
This is the only plan that has ever helped me achieve such an amazing result and make me feel confident about myself. I had got to a point where I had no motivation in completing any plan, simply because I wasn't getting much of a result. But this plan has changed my view of this because of the result I have had. I never feel hungry because the plan has helped create a routine for my meals. Instead of eating at irregular times like I used to, I now have breakfast, a snack, lunch, a snack and tea. My Mum and I enjoyed seeing the recipes posted by Christianne online to give us new ideas especially tasty snacks such as the energy bars, chocolate biscuits and cookies which are delicious if you have a sweet tooth!

From the start of the plan I was focused on what I wanted to achieve and maintained my willpower throughout in order to reach my goal. Part of my motivation was due to following the plan with my Mum which made the plan easier to follow during meal times, alongside inspiring one another. After completing the 12 week plan, I lost 23lbs which I am overwhelmed by, also my Mum lost an amazing 27lbs, so we both achieved an amazing result. The plan has had a big influence on our lifestyle and we shall both continue to follow the plan and try new recipes."
Saskia Allison

Mother & Daughter special!

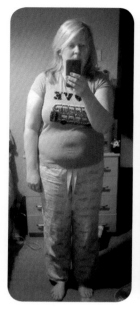 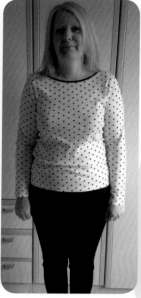 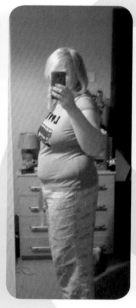 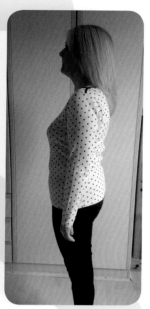

"I have tried low fat diets and fasting before but the weight just creeps back on. Seeing Catherine Huntley and how fab she looks, I decided to look into The Body Rescue Plan.

My daughter also wanted to lose a few pounds and change the way she was eating so we both decided to start the plan together at the beginning of March. We found it a lot easier than expected once getting over the first three days in which we had a bit of a headache.

I never enjoy cooking, I'm more of a baker however I actually enjoyed cooking during this plan. I make meals that I would have never made before and I also eat a lot more variety of vegetables and enjoy them.

So at the end of the 12 week plan I have lost 27lbs and my daughter has lost 23lbs. Not only have we lost weight but we feel so much better in ourselves and we plan to keep up with the healthy eating.

For me, there have been other positives resulting from following this plan. I sleep so much better at night and I don't have aching hip joints like I used to have each morning.

I love the way I feel and that is how I plan to continue."

Paula Allison

04: Testimonials

Find out from my clients how the Body Rescue Plan changed their lives.

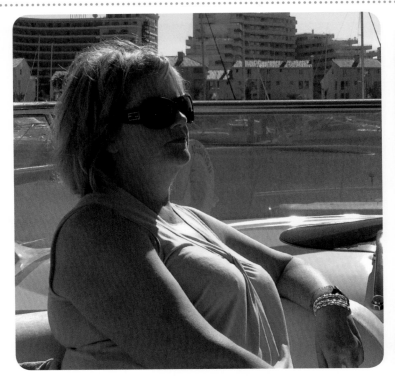

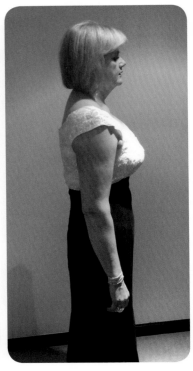

"I'm 53 years old and over the years I've yo yo dieted. I've done so many diets... weightwatchers/the F Plan/Herbal Life/Atkins to name but a few. And yes I lost weight. I would practically starve myself until "that special event" and once the event had passed I would relax and go back to good old Helen who ate and drank a lot. The "big girl" ...."great appetite" and that's how my life was. But when I did the diets I was tense, almost angry and fanatical. I just kept thinking don't worry when "the event" has passed it will be all over and when it was, there was almost a sense of relief. The trouble was I wouldn't just put some weight back on I would put it all back on...and more. To be honest I wasn't very happy. I also was pretty moody. On top form one moment and then snappy and argumentative the next. (My husband can vouch for this!)

But here I am sitting at home on Saturday 11th April 2015 the lightest, fittest and most content I have ever felt in my whole life. I have lost 1 stone 9lbs and I have dropped a good 2 dress sizes. And why? Because I went on The Body Rescue Plan.

As I'm writing this I actually feel quite emotional. I have never been in such a wonderful place before.

No this didn't happen overnight I have had to work at it .....but 12 weeks out of a whole life time is nothing.

When I thought about writing this piece I just kept asking myself how can I get it over to people that I am just an ordinary girl who has always liked her food and drink and that I never thought I could look or feel like this. And if I can do it PLEASE believe me when I say anyone can do it. To me Christianne is an angel on earth. She doesn't judge she is kind caring and hilarious! She knows we live ordinary busy lives so things need to be easy and simple to follow. What she has written and developed has worked for all sorts of people . This isn't a diet and this isn't just a book. This is truly a way of living and the principles of which I know I will follow for the rest of my life.

Yes the foods are delicious (especially the nut bread and curried lentils!) Yes the exercise programme is so easy to follow and makes you feel strong and fit but one aspect of the whole programme that has helped me enormously is the mind-set work.

Anyone can stop eating and lose weight. But to understand why you eat so much in the first place and to be aware of it ....well this is what takes this programme to another level for me. I now understand I eat too much to fill an emotional hole in me. I know I eat too much when I am tired or tense. But gradually over the last 12 weeks I have learnt this and I have learnt how to stop this self-sabotage and to believe in myself and want to care for myself.

I can honestly say this programme has changed my life.

The other thing I wanted to get across to people was that to begin with I thought about starting the programme but then I thought I can't as I've got a big dinner at work....I've got a family party...I'm going on a girls away trip...so I can't start until I have got a completely free diary. But as we know this isn't reality there is always something big or small that we can use as an excuse not to start. But Christiannes mind-set programme helped me to overcome these anxieties. I went to all the events, I followed the principles of the programme and after the event I felt stronger because of what I had achieved.

This programme is something anyone can follow. The food plan and recipes are so easy and so tasty. I haven't felt hungry. In fact some days I have struggled to eat everything! The exercise programme you can do anywhere ...at home or even in a hotel room (as I have done!).

This has been one of the most amazing journeys of my life and without Christianne I would never have experienced it. I wish everyone could have a Christianne in their lives and with this book or online you pretty much can! Trust her, believe in her as I have done and I can honestly say it will be the most wonderful experience.....it will be life changing.

Thank you Christianne xxxxxx"

Helen Burgess

04: Testimonials

Find out from my clients how the Body Rescue Plan changed their lives.

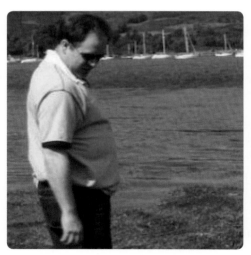
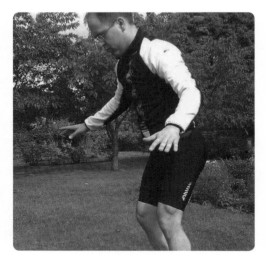

"When I started training with Christianne I had no real idea of the magnitude of the change I was beginning.

I went with the hope of losing some weight and having more energy. I didn't know how well it would work or even if it would work. Like many people, I'd just lost all motivation to try to lose weight and get fit. I'd tried gyms and diets but nothing seemed to work. There was always an excuse to avoid trying to eat better or exercise. And I was just getting fatter and more tired. With work becoming increasingly challenging, I reached a point where I felt I needed to have a big push (I think in my mind it might have been a last big push) to try to do something to improve my health. Christianne transformed my view of exercise, diet and what was possible. I lost 3 stone and 10 inches off my waist. I had to throw away almost all my clothes, but that was such a positive, cathartic change. I've found I get compliments on how good I look. Who knew my male friends were so aware of these things?! I'd thought I'd have trouble finding the

time to exercise, but miraculously, in taking time to work out, my work got better as my mental acuity improved as a result of the fitness. I became more effective and less tense.

Christianne's combination of resistance, cross training and yoga worked really well to keep everything varied, building up core strengths but also developing overall fitness.

I was thinking about having a goal to see just how far this new found health could take me. And I agreed to enter a triathlon. Which for the old me is nothing short of miraculous. But such is the confidence that my newfound form has given me. I feel I understand enough about exercise and diet to keep on developing my fitness and be able to participate in physical activities without fear of coming in a very poor last.

The experience has been nothing short of life changing."

**Paul Field
MD**

(Since Paul wrote this he has completed several triathlons and this year is going for an Ironman!)

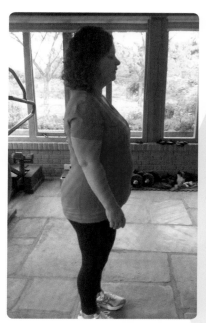 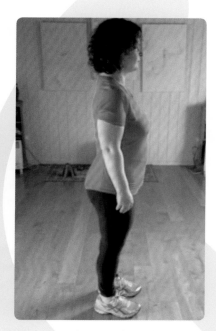

"Training with Christianne has had a profound impact for me. She has helped me to change lifelong eating habits and the way I see myself.

I now have an easily sustainable healthy diet that I really enjoy and shifts the pounds in a steady way. I am now lighter than I was when I got married nearly 20 years ago and have every confidence that I can achieve a physique that previously seemed completely impossible.

Christianne's method is particularly effective because she takes time to understand your circumstances; she also investigates mindset and motivation issues that could derail any progress. In my case I'm a busy, single working mother of three, which can be overwhelming.

Christianne doesn't make me feel bad if I have gone slightly off track with exercise due to this – she just helps me to work out what will work and methods to keep me motivated.

I particularly enjoy the variety of exercises that we do and always leave feeling uplifted and motivated.
I have now lost over 3 stone and am continuing to get fitter and leaner."

Nicola Atuyana

04: Testimonials

Find out from my clients how the Body Rescue Plan changed their lives.

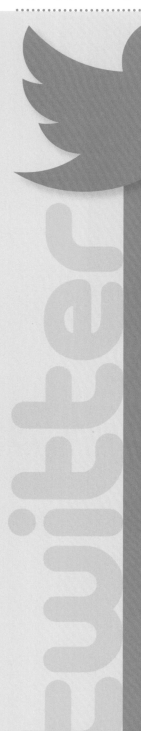

Taj phull @tajjy2011 · Feb 1

@Christianne_W week 3 starts and im already 11 lbs down. Come on the rescue plan.

   1 ⭐ 2 •••

Patsy Collyer @patsycollyer · 5h

@Christianne_W @TheHuntley Will do. Thank you! This plan is a revelation! :)

View conversation

 1   1 •••

Patsy Collyer @patsycollyer · 7h

@Christianne_W @TheHuntley Day 9 of the BRP detox and I'm forcing myself to eat. No hunger pangs whatsoever! :) x

  1   1 •••

Patsy Collyer @patsycollyer · 30m

@Christianne_W @TheHuntley Two weeks doing the detox and my 'tight' jeans are loose... Can't wait for week 12! thebodyrescueplan.com

 1   1 •••

Penni Rowe @sparkle0918 · 3h

@Christianne_W better than ever my partner and I have lost over 2 st put together & we're only in wk 6 we feel much healthier & energized x

View conversation

 1   1 •••

diannebarratt @diannebarratt · Feb 23

@TheHuntley @Christianne_W After following the body rescue plan I have lost a stone since Christmas. Both of you have been my inspiration xx

 1   1 •••

Gracie McLaven @graciemclaven · Feb 23

@Christianne_W - @AliMclaven and I have had a fab 1st week on the plan, both 8lbs lighter as well!

 1   1 •••

★★★★★ **Best Book Ever**

" 5 Stars and more for this book. I was a bread and butter girl along with chocolate bars but I am now a changed woman.

I have been following the book for two weeks and have lost 7lbs and I feel so much better and I am. so happy. I'm going away to the Canaries in March and I can't wait to wear my bikini.

I can't believe that I am so disciplined. Thank you Christianne you are amazing!!! "

★★★★★ **Love Body Rescue**

" this book is fab and easy to follow. Love the holistic process and easy to stick to. I never feel hungry and already lost over 2lbs in just 3 days. I WILL reach my goal.... Thank you all
Luv Shazzababes xx "

★★★★★ **Amazing**

" I'm now on week 3 and I feel really well,I'm also 9lbs lighter. This book is really easy to follow,I cant believe how I know longer crave chocolate and carbs. I can honestly say that I've never been hungry,and the dreaded heartburn and bloated and lethargic feeling has gone. I'm so glad that I bought this book. I'm so looking forward to the new slim me in the spring. "

★★★★★ **Totally amazing! Life changing!**

" I am in the 2nd week of the detox and am feeling amazing. This book (well to be honest it's far more than a book) is incredible. I am in my early 50's and over the years have calorie counted yo yo dieted and NOTHING has made me feel as good as this programme. The book is easy to follow but the mind set work is what is really helping me. I feel on a journey which is changing my life. So far I have list 6lbs but it's not just weight loss I'm looking for its a way of life I'm wanting.i have today made the nut bread on page 99 it's is so easy to make and is totally scrummy! I've had it with fresh mango on top and going to have bruschetta tomorrow!!! The exercises are also easy to follow. Christianne you are truly amazing thank you for changing my life I wish I had met you years ago! Helen xxx "

2 of 2 people found this review helpful.

Was this review helpful?   Yes | No   Share:

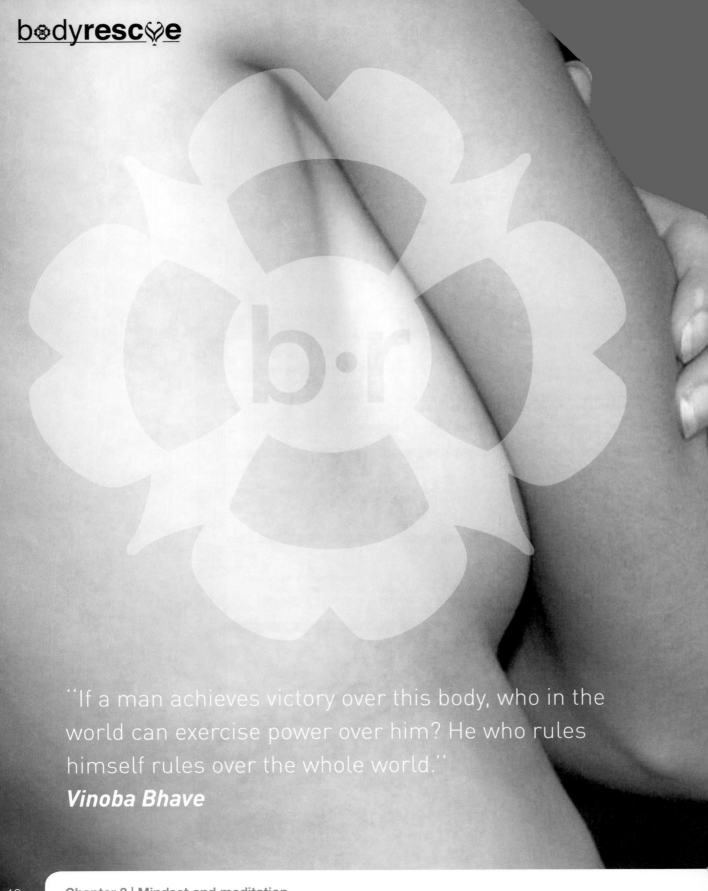

"If a man achieves victory over this body, who in the world can exercise power over him? He who rules himself rules over the whole world."

Vinoba Bhave

Chapter 3
Mindset and meditation

01: Goals

02: Desire statements

03: Language and willpower

04: Trigger points

05: Avoiding pain versus confronting fear

06: Unhealthy priorities

08: Guided meditations with visualisations

09: The Body Rescue Plan Meditations are..

10: Vision boarding

11: Gratitude

Mindset and meditation Introduction

I see endless exercise videos, fitness books, and nutritional plans all sold as 'the only way to lose weight', but
- **What happens when your enthusiasm dwindles?**
- **When you get stressed and there is no back-up plan?**
- **When you get tired and want to jack it in?**
- **Have you been there?**

Chances are you did jack it in, you did get bored and stop exercising, and you did get stressed and reach for the chocolate or bottle!

Well, I have some amazing ways in this chapter, that deal with all these issues and more, so that you will not screw it up again!

This chapter will be THE most important part of the plan, please read carefully as this is what will get you out of old habits and give you the ability to sustain this for the rest of your life. Being happier, younger, brighter, slimmer, and having an abundance of energy.

When I was a little girl, I really understood the power of the mindset and the control of the mind from a very young age. This was learnt through a combination of being brought up in a Catholic environment, being schooled in convents, and learning from my very large family, with older brothers.

Let me explain..
I was the youngest of five till I was eight years old, and then two more of my lovely siblings came along. Until then my brothers and sisters and I had endless play fights and, with me being the youngest, I was also the weakest. This left me with the need to be more powerful and to block out pain. The pain I am talking about is being tickled to death. My brothers and sisters would pin me down and tickle me till it was unbearably painful, I'm sure you have been there! One day I realised that if I played dead, closed my eyes and just shut out the noise, I wouldn't feel it more. I instantly stopped being ticklish and can do it to this day.

I adopted the same strategy when my fear of spiders became overwhelming. I used to scream out to my mum if one was in my bedroom at night (usually there were several, I was brought up in a large, 400 year old farm house in the country) and my wonderful mother would calmly come in with a cup, cover the spider and place it outside. I decided that after my tickling triumph I could get over my fear of spiders. I was right, I did! Our natural instinctive nature to be scared of spiders serves us well if we live near poisonous ones, but I live in the UK where they pose no threat, and therefore this fear did not serve me well – but being brought up in a house that had mice, silverfish, glis glis, and giant spiders was obviously something I needed to tolerate.

Meanwhile, one of my brothers sussed out I was a little scared of climbing our big oak tree right to the top. So he placed my favourite bracelet on the top branch of the tree and merrily went back to boarding school for two months! It either rusted up there or I had to save it. Again, I tapped into the same mindset, admittedly this was tinged with a desire to not be shamed when my brother made his return – I got to the top of that tree before the two months was up! This was the same will I had to use

when another brother held my feet in the swimming pool to teach me to swim, I either drown
swam, and so I swam. Don't get me wrong, I love my siblings dearly, they are my life – and tat
well – this was fun and banter and part of being in a big family; well, any sized family really.

My Catholic upbringing taught me a lot too – whilst I no longer am a practicing Catholic, the elements
I took from it and love are the power of prayer. At school and home we were taught to pray by saying
what you are thankful for (gratitude), saying sorry (ridding guilt), asking for help (goal focussing), and
having faith (power of the positive mind), and fundamentally these attributes make up the basis of my
mindset programme, as well as many other mindset programmes out there.
Big brothers, spiders and praying was the start of realising the power of the mind.

01: Goals

There are so many things I want to say to you about mindset, but I will start quite simply by asking ...

First things first – what is your goal?

I am going to ask you a series of questions to make sure you get some depth to this answer.
Please answer below..

How much weight do you want to lose?

What do you want to be your goal weight after 12 weeks on the programme?

What do you want your dress size to be?

**If you could choose a celebrity or other person, whose body do you think you could look like you
admire?** (to answer this make sure you choose someone that is your body shape, i.e.: pear, apple,
ruler etc., so don't choose Kate Moss if you are hourglass).

How much energy do you have now?

What body part would you most like to improve the look of?

How do you want to feel after the 12 weeks?

What clothes would you like to wear?

What activity would you like to do, that you do not do now because of how you look and feel?

How is your complexion?

How is your digestion?

Are you addicted to certain foods? (meaning you can't go a day or two without them – coffee, tea,
bread, alcohol and sugar/chocolate/biscuits are the usual culprits).

How attractive do you feel?

How attractive do you want to feel?

Do you feel light or heavy?

Do you currently exercise?I If so, how much effort are you putting into it?

How are your concentration levels?

Do you want better cognitive function?

Do you get tired at 3-4p.m?

Are you moody?

How are you sleeping?

Do you wake up feeling good in the morning?

Do you feel positive about life?

Is your libido low?

Is there anything else you would like to improve?

Take a before photo and place here.

Put your measurements here of your:

Waist

Hips

Chest

Thighs

What is your weight?

What do you want to be in 12 weeks?

What is your dress size?

What do you want it to be in 12 weeks?

Measure again at:

Week 4

Weight

Waist

Hips

Chest

Thighs

Week 8

Weight

Waist

Hips

Chest

Thighs

Week 12

Weight

Waist

Hips

Chest

Thighs

· ·

When you have finished place your after photo here and compare to the week 1 photo
- use this to continue your mindset thereafter.

The Body Rescue Plan will not only help you lose up to 2.5 stone in 12 weeks, but there are so many other ways it will improve your life. If you stick to it – your complexion will improve, your organs will function more efficiently, so that your metabolism works more effectively, you will be more hydrated, younger looking, your eyes will be brighter and bigger, your blood pressure will be lower, your pulse will be lower, you will have bags more energy, your moods will be nicer, you will be more toned and in shape, your fat percentage will lower, your dress size will lower, to name just a few..

02: Desire statements

So now I want you to summarise that goal into one sentence.
E.g.: I adore how it feels to be 2.5 stone lighter, so I have more energy, feel sexier, live longer, and can attract more things in my life through my clearer energy.

What's your sentence? (make it in the present tense, don't use words like I want to, I will, I am going to etc..)

_____

_____

_____

_____

The next step with your goal is to add a desire statement to it, so it helps you able to really visualise it more. Some people have so many negative attachments to being slim and losing weight, that they find it hard to visualise themselves as beautifully slim. These five statements will help you open your goal up more.

1. I have decided that ...
2. I love knowing that ...
3. It excites me that ...
4. I love how it feels when ...
5. I love seeing myself as ...

So you could say:
1. I have decided that I am losing 2.5 stone.
2. I love knowing that The Body Rescue plan is making me healthier and happier.
3. It excites me that every day I feel better and better.
4. I love how it feels when I wake up in the morning and am slimmer and fitter.
5. I love seeing myself as gorgeous and fit.

What are your statements? Please focus on how you feel as well as how you look.

_____

_____

_____

_____

_____

_____

_____

03: Language and willpower

Mindset is 90% of your success.

If you want to be in truly great shape, feel fantastic, have the energy of an athlete, have incredible willpower, look the best you can look, be calm, focussed and confident, it all starts with mindset. There are no two ways about it, mindset is the first thing you need to address if you are changing your routine to alter your body and mind.

First of all the language that you use will define who you are.
There is a Hebrew term, davar, which has a translation of 'You are what you speak'.

How you think will ultimately make you the person you are.
Do you see the negative in everything or the positive? Is the glass half-full or half-empty?

You are as capable as anyone else whatever your past is-
we all have different starts in life, but we all hear stories of people who have succeeded against all the odds; through their positive mind set they believe they can achieve anything, and through will they can.

Equally if your mindset is programmed to think you CANNOT do this, you WILL NOT do this, you shape your future- YOU!

Are you continually using limiting language on yourself?
For example:
* 'I have no confidence in going to a gym'
* 'I don't have the time to get fit'
* 'I'd never have the energy to live without sugar and caffeine'
* 'I don't have the patience for yoga and meditation'
* 'I'm too tired and stressed to change'
* 'It's not like I can do anything to make things better.'

These phrases are just a small part of how we limit ourselves every day. We are constantly negative about how we look, how we sound and who we are. So, with just the small sayings above make a conscious effort to change your language and thought patterns so that eventually your conscious becomes part of your subconscious and you automatically omit and attract positivity – you will be amazed at how quickly you can succeed in this.

So, for instance, the above quotes can be changed to:
* 'I am comfortable training in front of others, the more I workout the more confident I am'
* 'I have the time for getting fit because it is a priority'
* 'When my body is free from toxins I have abundant REAL energy'
* 'My mind is like a muscle, the more I use it to relax the calmer I feel'
* 'Change is exactly what I need to release the calm and energised me'
* 'I can always do something to make things better'

Language tends to reveal a lot about your subconscious beliefs. And someone listening closely to the words you use can tell a lot about you: are you a confident person or do you have low self-esteem?

Are you positive and optimistic or is everyone out to get you?

The important thing to remember is that you can also change your subconscious thinking patterns by changing how you speak. Just by making a few small changes you can increase your confidence and build your attraction muscles. Real change happens when you change your mindset, and you can change your mindset by changing the way you speak. When you catch yourself using negative words, rephrase your sentence and try again. Becoming more aware of your language is the first step towards change. Enjoy how it feels to be more positive ... and keep telling yourself, 'I can do it!'

04: Trigger points

The next step to my mindset plan is to figure out what your trigger points are in eating too much or eating something that you know doesn't agree with you.

Trigger points can be anything that makes you eat without actually being hungry.

The following trigger points for eating too much or eating junk food with my clients are usually:
(Tick what applies to you.)

I eat when I am stressed

I eat when I am happy and want to celebrate

I eat when I am lonely

I eat when I am depressed

I eat when I am nervous

I eat when I am tired

I eat when I am bored

I eat for something to do

I eat the wrong thing through lack of organisation

I eat to punish myself/self sabotage

Please do add your reasons here for eating too much or tick the above and expand.

I have devised some meditation recordings especially for you with these trigger points, you can choose to use them every morning or every evening, which will work your willpower muscles every day, but you can also use them if you are confronted by something very stressful that is out of the norm, that makes these trigger points arise.

Trigger points can also be something else entirely ... for me, I feel hungry the moment I walk into my parents' house. They have an enormous kitchen, and I am one of seven children, so I have a natural tendency to want to eat to compete with my siblings for food. I also have a trigger point when I drive past petrol stations, I know the naughties that are inside and if I am having an off day I am tempted. Or even something as simple as feeling an old chocolate wrapper in your coat pocket can make you want to eat chocolate, just that rustle of the paper itself, or advertisements can easily entice you.

You may also have trigger points about not wanting to exercise or follow the meditations. The usual trigger points or excuses are:

- I am too tired to exercise
- I don't have the time
- I feel too depressed
- I feel too stressed

What are your trigger points for not wanting to exercise or meditate?

_____

_____

_____

_____

_____

Once you realise what your trigger points are you can really tune into them, so when you feel like eating, you can ask yourself 'Am I actually hungry, or am I responding to a trigger point?' If you then know what the trigger point is, you can confront it and ask it to go away (or use my meditation techniques).
This is incredibly empowering, knowing what is making you eat too much and having the power to stop it controlling you.

I often find with my clients, and with myself, that the pain of being hungry in your stomach versus the pain of being stressed in your stomach, are virtually the same feeling. Therefore when you are stressed and you feel it in your stomach you automatically want to eat, to stop that pain. So when you get that signal, stop and think – am I actually hungry or am I stressed ?(or bored or anything else) and if you are stressed, take some deep breaths, have a herbal tea or go for a walk and see if the feeling subsides.

The same goes with exercise, or food shopping, or cooking, or anything that is part of this programme, if you are not practicing it, is it genuinely for a legitimate reason? Or are you just responding to a trigger point?

Often we do not realise we are stressed, or eating out of boredom, or eating out of celebration.

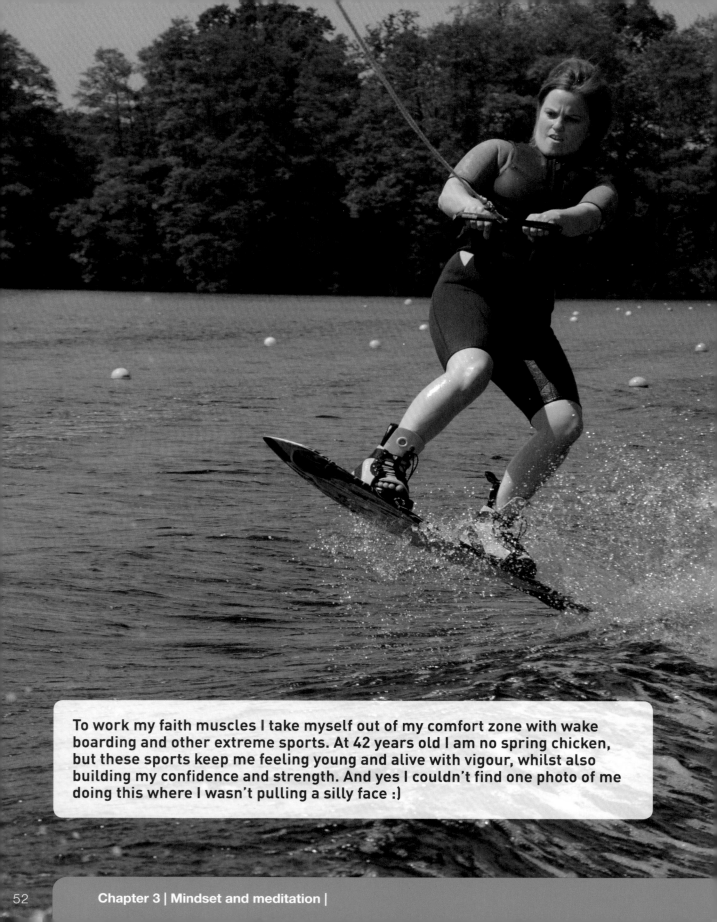

To work my faith muscles I take myself out of my comfort zone with wake boarding and other extreme sports. At 42 years old I am no spring chicken, but these sports keep me feeling young and alive with vigour, whilst also building my confidence and strength. And yes I couldn't find one photo of me doing this where I wasn't pulling a silly face :)

05: Avoiding pain/ confronting your fear

We associate foods with so many different things. If you think about all the religious festivals, they involve food and alcohol, particularly sweet foods – chocolates. We eat and drink at parties and birthdays and we also are given chocolate foods as a prize when we are younger or as a bribe. We are used to using foods as comfort and celebration.

Did you know that using foods for comfort is our oldest primal instinct?

Have you ever noticed that when you write your list of things to do that day or that week, you avoid tackling the more difficult ones till last?

Or have you noticed that the all-important phone call you need to make goes on the back burner, because you do the' nice' things first?

We call this procrastination, but actually it's one of our oldest survival instincts!

In order to survive, our bodies respond to avoid pain as a healing mechanism.

As we feel hunger or thirst, our instinct is to obviously eat or drink
 – to avoid the pain our body will endure through starvation and thirst, and subsequently death!

In order to avoid breaking a limb, or killing ourselves, we know to avoid anything that may cause us bodily harm – or it will damn well hurt!
But did you know that mentally we do this also?

Most humans will do anything to avoid pain; instinctively, we feel that pain will cause more pain, and so we procrastinate the painful tasks whilst doing the 'nice' things to avoid that pain.

Of course this is very helpful to avoid death, but it is also very unhelpful, especially when you are confronted with getting things done that feel uncomfortable to do. We seem to want instant gratification.

Many of my personal training clients suffer with this avoidance of pain when they first come to me, the fear of exercise and sticking to a healthy eating programme seems so utterly alien, or just a bit too painful even to face, let alone endure. But actually it's usually a fear of nothing but just a new thing.

That fear of doing something new is in most of us – as I said, it is instinctive and we also have a lovely ego that tells us that 'what we know already is far easier than something new'!

Luckily we can overcome this!
How?

By confronting our fears head on ...

First of all break it down – what are you scared of? Normally very little!

Now see yourself a year from now if you did not do that new thing
– i.e. your new fitness and nutrition programme – what do you see??

Now see yourself a year from now if you did do that new thing
– what do you see??

Obviously if we are in need of grabbing the bull by the horns now, and we don't, in a year's time our life will be a lot more painful – it will be harder to lose weight and get fit, we may feel more sore in our joints, we may get injuries more easily and our self-esteem will be lowered.

If we endured that first hurdle of realising the pain of doing a new thing, then this will get us a beautiful new body, loads of energy, and more confidence and health.

In order to do this we have to make doing something 'new' as part of our weekly or even daily tasks, so that we associate them not with pain, but with excitement and happiness and moving up to the next level :)

Give a positive prize like a child
– when you do these new tasks give yourself a prize of some sort that does not involve food!

So give yourself a little task today of things you are avoiding on your to do list
– ask yourself why you are not doing them and then see the results if you do or do not do them. AND THEN DO THEM! One step at a time.

And if you are used to eating out of comfort to dull a pain, why not offer yourself a prize if you exercise and stick to the eating plan, but something that is not food
Put money in a jar for every day you stick to it and face your pain, and buy yourself something that will make you feel amazing.

....

What I also like to do with myself and my clients, is do things out of our comfort zone. By doing this you are achieving so much more than just that scary task at hand. You are educating your brain and body to push the limits, to be happy and excited by the new and different and to enjoy the challenge rather than avoid it.

What will you do thats out of your comfort zone?
(It doesn't have to be something big to begin with, but gradually let it build each week)

06: Unhealthy priorities

We all have unhealthy priorities in our life that really make no sense at all.

I have had many clients sit in front of me with obesity, or high blood pressure, or chronic back pain caused by lack of movement, and yet their priorities are obsessively cleaning, or having a pristine car or making a lot of money at the cost of their health and home life.

Isn't it funny what we prioritise when if we really think about it, it makes no sense at all? And when does that priority turn into a habit, and then an obsession and finally an addiction?

Habits are easier to make than they are to break and if you repeat a behaviour often enough, our brain's synaptic pathways are going to get broken in as the human brain is a very adaptive piece of machinery. Breaking a habit is a lot more complicated, because while parts of those worn-in pathways can weaken without use, they never go away. With the slightest provocation they can be reactivated.

If you've ever tried to quit smoking, you already know this. You can go a year without a cigarette, and then give in one time and the habit can come right back.

The way to break a habit is to form a new, parallel pattern, like exercising when you feel stress, rather than indulge the old pattern, which triggers 'cigarette' in response to stress.

When I was over weight, whenever I was stressed I would eat, without even realising it. Now when I get that anxious feeling I either take my self out for a walk , focus on my breath or meditate- because I have trained myself that the out come of that will make me feel much better and the out come of gorging on food will not- in fact I usually felt worse!

So think about what you should make your priority,

and for every unhealthy habit make a healthy one!

And remember, it can take six weeks to make a habit and two days to break it!

07: Limiting beliefs

As part of the mindset programme in The Body Rescue plan, I have recorded 6 meditations for you but before you do the visualisations I would like you to perform a task which highlights what your self-limiting beliefs are. These are what you believe you should do, or be, your expectations about yourself.

Do you have any beliefs that could act as self sabotage for new slim you?
Really think about this. Imagine yourself slim, and in every scenario – meeting people, seeing friends, family, at work – is there anything that does not feel right? If so, write it down and work with that.

What is the conflict that is holding you back? What limiting beliefs do you have about yourself that is tarnishing this? This is important to really grasp before anything else as if you do not confront your limiting beliefs now, they will come back in the future to sabotage your success.

You may find that once you become sensitive to your own limiting beliefs and change your thoughts and language you will notice it in others too. Be a guide to others to change their thought patterns, it is important for your own confidence and self esteem that you surround yourself with positive people. Negative people will pull you down, they will not want you to succeed, so either help them change or move away from them.

Please write your limiting beliefs here.
My clients' typical limiting beliefs are that they have tried many diets before and they only work for a few weeks and then their lack of willpower kicks in, so they feel they are going to fail. Ultimately this a fear of failure, which is very significant.
- You may be thinking the detox will be too hard (it won't, you will be fine).
- You may have friends and family that are unsupportive when you get slimmer and want to feed you.
- You may have drinking friends who won't support you whilst you are going through a cleanse.
- You may feel you don't have enough time.

What are your limiting beliefs about sustaining my 12 week plan?

The next step is to allow these limiting beliefs to not be part of you anymore.
We do this with my very powerful visualisations that picture you with your limiting beliefs and then as the powerful you alone. These visualisations are really important, you may be feeling really confident and excited about starting this programme now, but after a few weeks your old limiting beliefs may kick in, you know, the ones that have stopped you achieving your dreams in the past, so if you have these mental exercises in place, they will protect you from old past habits.

08: Visualisation and guided imagery

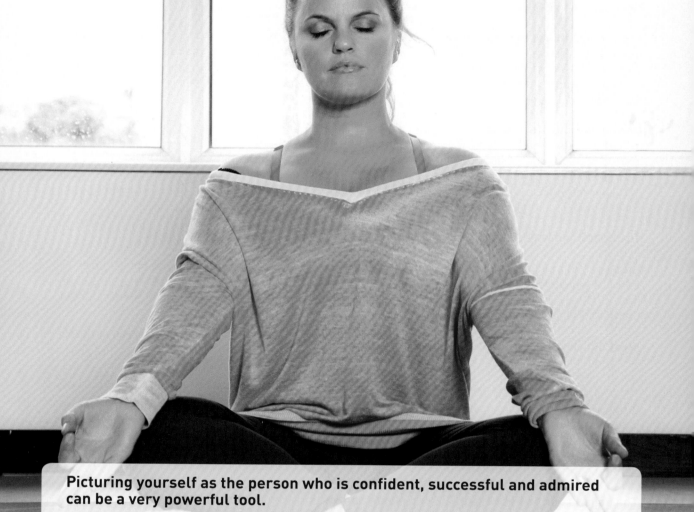

Picturing yourself as the person who is confident, successful and admired can be a very powerful tool.

If you can believe it, you can achieve it.

Our conscious mind accounts for about 10% of our functioning; the other 90% of your mind controls the rest of you!

Our minds can effect physiological changes in our bodies just by using thought. In sports, we see people change the degree of their performance through mind control, by visualising the win. The UK javelin champion, Steve Backeley, used visualisation whilst he was in plaster from an injury. He regularly practiced throwing the javelin in his mind, through visualisation, and when the plaster was removed his muscle had only shrunk slightly, to the great surprise of his doctors.

The body cannot tell the difference between imagined situations and real life. If you think ahead to when you have to do an exam you can get physical anxiety symptoms weeks before, or if you watch a horror movie your hair may stand on end and or your heart may beat faster, or your body can have a sexual response to something you imagine!

This is also how placebo works and some forms of hypnosis and meditation. The power of your mind is enormous and can be both positive and detrimental, depending on how you choose to use it. The same forces that imprison you can also empower you.

You can use things to help you visualise too- I bought a lovely Karen Millen little black cocktail dress three weeks before my birthday - it was too tight but was a bargain, so I just had to have it! I tried it on every other day, and it slowly was getting there, so when I did my visualisations I visualised it fitting perfectly. I wanted to look the best I could for hitting forty, so I didn't have a mid-life crisis. And it looked fab for the day!

Do you have an old item of clothing you can do this with? Or are you prepared to go out and buy one item that is too small? This really helps with visualising. But please don't start wearing clothes that are too small as that is not good for the morale, just one item will do that you keep trying on and seeing yourself in. Some people find visualising themselves as slim really difficult, so this method of actually wearing an item of clothing and then picturing it fitting can be easier. Especially when you see yourself looking slimmer in it each week as you try it on.

To understand why visualising is really powerful, please read the next paragraph...

I want you to imagine you are going into your kitchen, and you walk towards your chopping board. You take out a big juicy lemon from your fruit bowl and place it on your board. You then take out a sharp knife and cut into the zesty lemon. As you cut into it you see some of the juice fly out. Then, you hold the lemon up to your mouth and squeeze...

What did you notice happened when you visualised this?
You should have salivated – this is your physical response to your visualisation.

．．．

When we visualise things, our brain can't distinguish between what is real and what's not, when it comes to our physical response. The same goes for when we see a scary film, our hair can stand on end, our heart can beat faster, or if we read something emotional, we can cry or get a lump in the throat, even if it is fantasy, or the same goes for something that makes us laugh or even a sexual response to something arousing!!!

The point is our bodies respond to our minds' thoughts, and so when you visualise your body as slimmer, positive and happy, and when you say your positive mantra, your body will have a physical response by getting slimmer. I promise you this works. In the same respect, if you feel negative about your body and don't believe you can ever get the body you want, you never will.

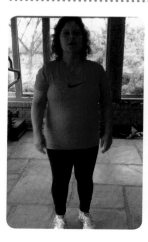
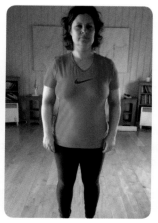
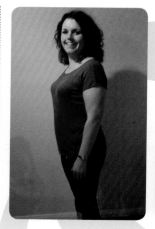
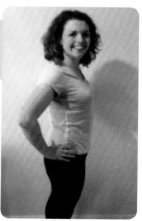

I did this with my client Nicola, photos above, and she was a size 18 (UK size) when we started.

On day one, I asked her:
'Where do you want to be in ten weeks?'
Nicola screwed up her face and replied hesitantly,
'A size 14?'

She said it with no determination and did not believe it.
I said that actually I thought she would get to a size 12 in ten weeks, and she looked at me with total disbelief.

So for the first week we did loads of positive visualisations to help her see that actually it is possible to see her figure at a size 12. After one week she could really visualise it and did so every day.

And guess what? She has gone from a size 18 to a size 12 in ten weeks!

And if she can do it so can you – she is run off her feet busy, a single mum of three, she works full time and can still fit in the time for herself, and by doing so she has so much more energy now for herself. Her life has been transformed.

Another client of mine, Mernie Gilmore, Women's Editor of The Daily Express, found it difficult to visualise herself as a size 12.

It took one and a half weeks and then we got there. She found it easier to visualise her before and after photos, like my client's photos above, and to understand that if they did it she can do it, too, as they followed exactly the same plan as she is doing.

''You should sit in meditation for twenty minutes every day, unless you are too busy?

In which case you should meditate for two hours.''

Zen proverb

09: Guided meditations with visualisations

There are six guided meditations that come with this book, each is to guide you through any issues and old habits you may have, and to reinforce you onto new healthy habits. To download your audio meditations please go to www.thebodyrescueplan.com.

You can choose to do one meditation a day, which covers six days a week, and have one day off. Or if there is one you particularly resonate with or feel is the burning issue to your weight loss problems, then stick with that one for a while.

Do try all of the meditations, though, as you may not realise how powerful they actually are.

For your convenience they are only ten minutes each; ideally it would be great for you to extend that to twenty minutes, so if you have time, just allow some silence at the end of the meditation.

Over the last seventeen years of teaching meditation to my clients I have found the six meditations below to be the main issues that are behind all my clients' weight loss problems.

1.   **Goals, limiting beliefs and seeing yourself at the place you want to be**
2.   **Working the faith muscle and ridding fear**
3.   **Ridding guilt**
4.   **Self-sabotage/devil in your head**
5.   **Greed**
6.   **Stress**

*   **It could be that you are riddled with guilt, and eat or don't exercise or punish yourself in some unhealthy way.**
*   **It could be you have a lack of self-worth and self-sabotage.**
*   **It could be you have an overwhelming urge to eat/are addicted, which we call greed.**
*   **It may be that just simply de-stressing yourself is the simplest one to use for you as you always eat under stress.**
*   **It could be that you have a fear of letting go of something from the past that is linked with eating.**
*   **It could be that you do not trust yourself to sustain this.**

-The main one I want you to make sure you do every week is focus on your goals – this one really works its magic, without you even knowing it.

··

I often find my clients' reactions interesting when confronted with visualisations and meditations. My clients may say...

'How can focussing on a goal or being positive about something possibly lead to weight loss or a fitter body, or attracting something good in your life?'
But then in the same breath they would say...

'I don't want to focus on the weight loss goal because I might jinx it.'

So on the one hand they are saying that mindset and thought could not possibly react to create an outcome, and then on the other hand they are saying if they think positively about something it will have an outcome, but a negative one!

Everything is connected and the more you work with the mind, the more you realise that the tiniest of thoughts leads to a butterfly effect – which is the phenomenon whereby a minute localised change in a complex system can have large effects elsewhere, even a typhoon!

··

We can also often not realise what we are reacting to, or when we are stressed.
An example of this is when we drive on long journeys. I know that if I drive for more than an hour, I want to eat – which is ridiculous, as if I am just at home for an hour, or working for an hour, I do not have the desire to eat. But driving, there are a few things going on.

1. I think I am relaxed, but actually there are so many things going on that my brain has to focus on, I am actually stressed and therefore my old habits of wanting to eat when I am stressed are coming in to play

2. I am programmed from a young age that a long car journey leads to eating yummy sweets; when I was young we always had those boiled sweets in a beautiful tin for long car journeys.

3. I get bored, and again my old instilled habits of eating to ease the 'pain of boredom'.

This is just one example where most people are totally un-mindful of what's actually going on inside them. They probably do not realise they are stressed, bored and triggering childhood eating patterns, but this kind of subconscious thought pattern is triggered in us every day, particularly if we are very focussed on something else like driving.

10: The Body Rescue Plan Meditations are...

1. **Goals, limiting beliefs and seeing yourself at the place you want to be**
2. **Working the faith muscles/ridding fears**
3. **Ridding guilt**
4. **Self-sabotage/devil in your head**
5. **Greed**
6. **Stress**

To download your audio meditations please go to www.thebodyrescueplan.com adding the code TBRP1..

1 Meditation for Goals

This meditation is about going back to your limiting beliefs and goal setting and focussing on the end goal, absorbing your energies into what it's actually like to feel and look like you want to after the 12 weeks, so that your mind actually starts to believe it is happening right now.

2 Working the faith muscles/ridding fears

This meditation is about confronting what is actually going on in your subconscious when you face something you fear and the feelings that get stirred inside of you. It also highlights what your fears are, as often we do not realise because we eat to mask the fear. Then we release this fear and replace it with something more tangible and positive. I also work on helping you build your faith muscles so that you believe you can achieve this.

3 Ridding guilt

In this meditation I use a beautiful traditional Hawaiian meditation called Ho-oponopono – which has a mantra: 'I am sorry, please forgive me, I love you and I thank you'. I can't tell you how powerful this is. If you are someone that suffers with guilt and eats through guilt, this is so wonderful. It is also really good to use even if you are out and about, and you get glimmers of guilt in your mind, just say it in your mind and let that thought go.

4 Self-sabotage/devil in your head

I think we all suffer with that conversation in the head of our old ego telling us to 'have one, it won't hurt', or 'don't bother training, it can wait'. And often, just by creating a new habit we can rectify this conversation. But if you have a history of self-sabotage, even if you have religiously stuck to The Body Rescue Plan, that devil in your head can crop up at any point, particularly under stress. So this meditation really gets to grips with nurturing that self-infliction, healing it and letting it go.

5 Greed

I don't think there is such a thing as greed, it doesn't come from a nowhere selfish land, and is often born of addictive behaviour or masking a pain. So this meditation is understanding your so called greed, of how it manifests and again letting it go.

6 Stress
Relaxation will be THE best way to turn off your need to fail this plan. This meditation will make you feel like you have had a radiant bath and been on holiday for a week!

....

Making a plan
I would say the number one reason that my clients (prior to working with me) have stopped and started an exercise and eating regime, and therefore not reached their goal, is because there has been an interruption to their routine and they have not put measures in place to cope with that interruption.

Have you done this in the past?
So be it an emotional turmoil, illness, a business trip, a holiday, a weekend away, a meal out, a night out drinking, or even just a row with a friend or colleague – all these situations upset our routine and I bet you the first thing to suffer is your eating or your fitness. (Again, priorities!)

....

Being healthy is a really important part of your life and if you have not got control over anything in your life the one thing you can control is what you put in your mouth and sticking to your exercise routine.

As I wrote about my client Nicola, we have devised a system where you can rewrite your diary for every eventuality. If your routine has been affected by the above then look at your diary again and rewrite where you are going to fit your exercise and nutrition plan in. It is that simple, so stop living a bipolar lifestyle and stick to it. Treat The Body Rescue exercise, mindset and eating plan like it's a client that you have to make a meeting with in your diary, and nothing should interrupt that!

Being organised is important to begin with, as if exercise and eating well are not your priority then they never will be if you don't sit down and organise when and where you are going to fit them in. Eventually it may become second nature, but for now put in your diary when you are going to make your food, eat it, exercise and meditate.

Also, stock up all your cupboards full of healthy goodies, clear out any junk food – give it to food banks! Give your kitchen a de-clutter and completely blitz clean it.

....

Food diary
Please see chapter 10 with your food diary and exercise diary plan, or go to http://www.thebodyrescueplan.com/wp-content/uploads/2015/03/BR-Weekly-Plan.pdf for your print out version.

11: Vision boarding

What happens to your life when you are slimmer, fitter and full of energy, and looking hot! What are you attracting??

Will you be able to do something you haven't done before?

Will you be fitting into some amazing style clothes that previously you could not?

We always get confidence when we are more comfortable in our skin, where will that take you?

Vision boarding can be really powerful because you are looking at an image and absorbing the energy from it, it's like a fantastic aid to your visualisations and particularly useful if you are not able to visualise very well.

How to make a vision board

A vision board is simply a board on which you paste images and words that resonate with what you want to draw in. This then helps you focus your intention, which in turn raises your vibration, because it puts you in a brilliant mood every time you look at it.
You can spend an hour or two playing around with scissors, glue and magazines or even paint the scene yourself. If you would prefer to do it via the computer, social media sites like Pinterest enable you to make your own vision board.

If you want to make your own vision board, work along the following lines:

1) Look around to find images that you feel totally represent whatever it is you want to attract.
Look back to your goals list, maybe you have always wanted to do a particular sport but had to stop or never started due to your fitness levels. Maybe you want a gorgeous partner to share your life with, perhaps you want to go travelling but never dare reveal yourself on a beach. Find pictures that encompass this. You could even put an old slimmer photo of you on there.

2) You can also include single words or phrases,
such as 'love', 'abundance' or 'I feel great' that pack a powerful emotional punch. Or, if you look at the picture of my vision board, I have words like 'power' and 'lean'.

3) Make the process of putting it all together as magical as possible.
Light candles, put on music that lifts your spirits, and make sure you spend loads of time daydreaming about how amazing your life is going to be as all of this comes in as you put it together. You can even listen to my meditation CDs as you do this.

Create something that lifts and inspires you every time that you look at it.
If you don't feel comfortable with anyone in your house seeing it, take a photo on your phone and have it as your screen saver, or upload it to your computer, and look at it each day, envisioning your new and bright future.

My vision board

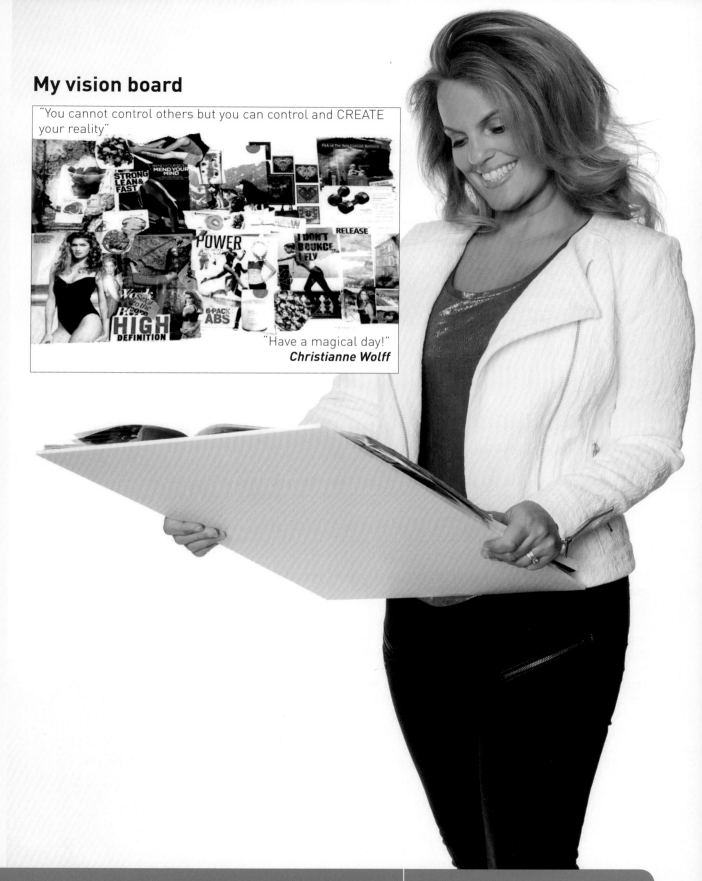

"You cannot control others but you can control and CREATE your reality"

STRONG LEAN & FAST

MEND YOUR MIND

POWER

RELEASE

I DON'T BOUNCE I FLY

HIGH DEFINITION

6-PACK ABS

"Have a magical day!"
Christianne Wolff

12 : Gratitude

When you start a new diet, or exercise regime, part of your mindset is probably thinking about what you are missing out on. This can be the very reason you give up, because you are being lured into the darker side, you know that side?

- **That thinks you won't have so much fun if you continue eating so well,**
- **That side that says you can only have fun if you get drunk,**
- **That side that says you can only be alert if you drink coffee,**
- **That side that says you are being a bore by looking after yourself.**

As a nation in the west we are really spoilt, we get used to the hundreds of food choices we have and feel we are well deserved to eat and drink what we so please.

Actually, there are some people in this world that would kill to eat like we would eat on my detox, or my eating plan, but to us we feel we are missing out somehow. With that in mind it is such a good idea to write a gratitude diary, to first of all appreciate the little things in life, that make the bigger picture amazing, but when you focus your attention on the positives in your life, you start attracting more and more.

I love this quote by Tom Hanks

"Eating everything you want is not that much fun. When you live a life with no boundaries, there's less joy. If you can eat anything you want to, what's the fun in eating anything you want to?"

What I would like you to do as part of this plan is to write a gratitude diary, this has been added into your diary in the last chapter.
You will be introduced to new foods, a new feeling to life, new energy and many other positives, so I want you to write down each day everything you find amazing, whether it's a new breakthrough, the food you ate, the energy you feel, the love you have for life, the new exercise you tried and how good that made you feel. By reinforcing this, it will become part of you.

And lastly, start having positive associations with all these new and exciting things you are trying.
Connect with this book, the cover, my name, the book's name, your notes inside it, even the dog ears you make and the stains on the book, everything about this book is improving your life, literally feel those vibrations through the feel, sight, sound and smell of the book.

I want you to feel my support every time you pick this book up, my love and compassion for you,
I am there for you, I know exactly what you are going through and I know you can get through this and swap the life that is not serving you for a life that will serve you.

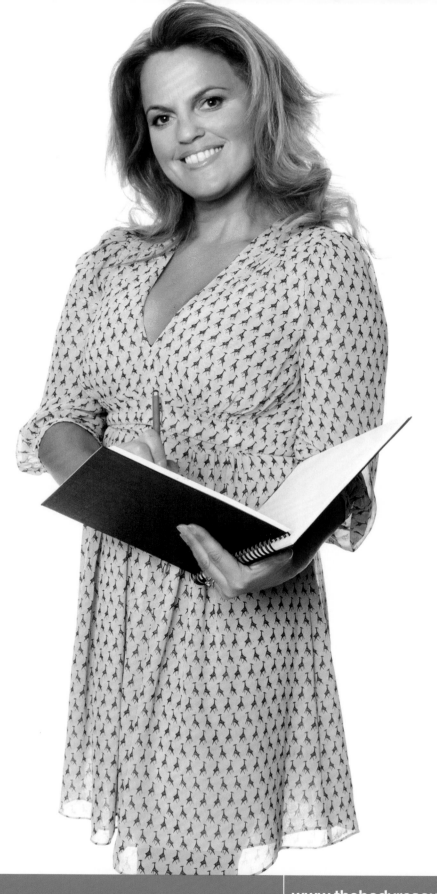

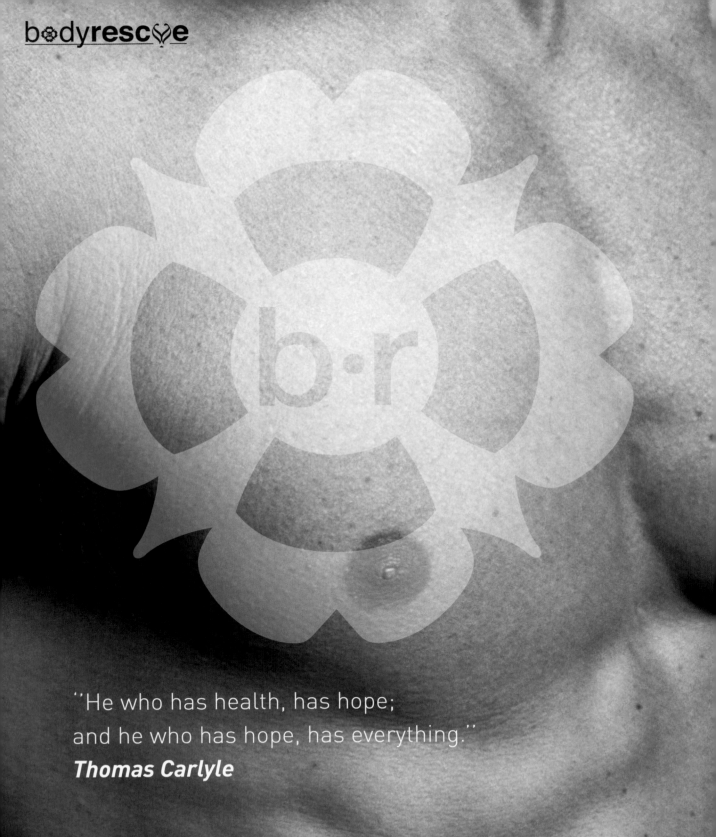

bodyrescue

"He who has health, has hope;
and he who has hope, has everything."
Thomas Carlyle

Chapter 4
Why Detox?

01: How to detox

02: Wheat and gluten

03: Dairy

04: Alcohol

05: Sugar

06: Other reasons to detox

07: Bath products

08: Other products

09: Foods that help a detox

10: Supplements and foods that can help you in a detoxification

11: Foods to avoid to cut belly fat

12: Sleep

13: Water

Part of the 11 golden rules of The Body Rescue Plan is detoxing

Our bodies naturally go through a detox process every day, by eliminating and neutralising toxins through the colon, liver, kidneys, lungs, lymph and skin.
In this day and age our bodies have a hard time keeping up with the polluted air we breathe, water we drink and food we eat. Our beautiful internal eco system has been radically changed through our chemicalised diet with, too much animal protein, too much saturated and trans fats, and too much caffeine, sugar and alcohol.

Our poor organs that were once capable of cleaning out unwanted substances are now completely over-loaded to the point where toxic material remains inside our tissues.

A special detoxing and cleansing diet is a good way to assist your body in its over-loaded state.
Even if your diet is normally good, an internal clean can revitalise your system and rid your body of harmful bacteria, viruses and parasites.

If your body is sluggish and over-burdened with toxicity, not only your ability to be motivated to lose weight could be hampered, but also your body's ability to shed the pounds could be seriously affected.

Stress can also impact your toxicity levels,
which is why included in The Body Rescue plan is exercise, meditation and yoga; to help cleanse your internal organs and uplift your mood.

Pollution is also another factor increasing your chances of being more consumed with toxins, so regular skin brushing, hot baths, saunas, and sweating all help, as well as getting out in the country and breathing in fresh air regularly.

01: How to detox

I love a good detox and am in my second week of one now;
it makes you feel lighter, more energised, less addictive, and more in control of foods.

With my Body Rescue Detox System I advise my clients to cut out:

- **Wheat and gluten**
- **Dairy**
- **Alcohol**
- **Sugar**
- **Caffeine**
- **Processed foods**

The idea behind this is to remove all toxins that are stored within the adipose fat cells, once these toxins are removed it then becomes easier to shrink your fat.

It is really important you stick to the detox, fully. You cannot have a day off, it does not work like that. I really need you to focus 100% on this.

You will feel amazing, very soon, so keep telling yourself that. Detoxing is designed to clear out toxins from your body so that your body works more efficiently. Your liver and colon do most of the clearing out and if they are cleansed, then they will work better. Your liver controls how many calories you burn a day, so if it's in top working order without having to slug along dealing with the crap you put in it, then your metabolism will be on fire.

Indulging in foods full of toxins does not give our cells the nutrients needed,
so the body sends a signal to consume more until its nutrition need is met. We eat to feed our cells, giving them the correct nutrition to grow and repair, and without the correct nutrients the body becomes diseased.

02: Wheat and gluten

Wheat has little nutritional value and digestion of both wheat and gluten is exceptionally difficult; chances are you will be intolerant to both wheat and gluten and not even realise – bloating, headaches, tiredness, are common side effects of gluten.

You may think you eat healthily but do you still feel bloated, tired and overweight?
Perhaps your diet is something like this:
- **You wake up in the morning and have a so called healthy cereal, or some toast.**
- **For lunch you have noodles or a healthy sandwich.**
- **Afternoon you have a snack of some dried biscuits, or maybe the odd naughty biscuit, but not too much as you are careful.**
- **Supper, you have a nice bowl of pasta with plenty of veg. Great, right?**

So, why are you feeling lethargic and bloated?
Because every single meal you are having has wheat in it and even if you were not naturally wheat intolerant you will build up an intolerance with the amount of wheat in your diet.

More and more people are discovering eliminating wheat from the diet brings positive results.
That is especially true if you realise you suffer from an intolerance to gluten (a grain protein). Symptoms can be psoriasis, migraine headaches to heart disease and arthritis.

So why is wheat intolerance such so prevalent in this day and age?
The wheat we eat today has been so processed it barely resembles the wheat of our ancestors. If gluten goes undigested, it causes problems both in the gut and in the bloodstream. This change may be caused by toxicity in our environment and the food chain.

Consuming grain was also never part of our make-up. As humans, we only started farming 10,000 years ago, yet we have had hundreds of millions of years as hunter-gatherers.

Whatever the cause, avoiding wheat or gluten seems to be a positive change everyone can make to their diets. I've personally witnessed my clients' health improve dramatically through this small change.

There is always a wheat-free bread, wheat-free pasta, wheat-free biscuits.
Just get to your health food shop and try. Or why not make my Nut bread on Chapter 7, page 109.

03: Dairy

If you are wondering where to get your calcium from without milk and cheese, you can actually get all you need from green vegetables, the darker the better. Nuts are also a fantastic source of calcium, almonds in particular. Cow's milk is good for you if you are a calf, but we do not have the same digestive system as a cow and therefore it is not beneficial to us. During pasteurisation many enzymes are destroyed, as well as vitamins and good bacteria.

Countries with the lowest rate of dairy consumption (Africa and Asia) have the lowest rate of osteoporosis, and the countries that take in the biggest consumption of dairy (America and the UK) have the highest rate of osteoporosis. Other good foods for bones are found high in Vitamin D.

04: Alcohol

Alcohol is a liquid sugar and does not hold any nutritional value to the body. The body has a huge release of insulin when drinking alcohol, which then informs your body there is a mass of energy available within the body, so the body stops burning fat and retains fat instead.

05: Sugar

Sugar is highly addictive and has no nutritional value to the body.
All it will do for you is contribute to an enormous amount of today's illnesses, including diabetes, and weight gain. Research has shown that sugar acts on the brain the same way as class A drugs do.

Sugar raises serotonin levels, which makes us feels good, when that starts to wear off we want more.

- **Are you stressed?**
- **Fat?**
- **Sleep badly?**
- **Have mood swings and or depression?**

Sugar can have this effect on your body, are you addicted?

Fructose or sucrose (table sugar) leads to high blood pressure, heart disease or diabetes.

High fructose corn syrup leads to diabetes, high blood pressure, liver disease, kidney disease, and vascular disease.

Eating whole fruits does not cause the same problem as high fructose corn syrup and table sugar, because the fruits contain vitamins, minerals, and antioxidants which help metabolise the fructose.

Some of the other effects of sugar on the body are:
- Chronic fatigue.
- Weight gain.
- Anxiety and irritability.
- Tooth decay.
- PMS symptoms.
- High blood pressure.

For every molecule of sugar you consume, it takes 54 molecules of magnesium to process it!

Reduce sugar cravings by...

-Eating protein and vegetables.
-Taking B vitamins.
-Taking chromium and magnesium.
-Getting 8 hours sleep a night.
-Drinking liquorice tea.
-Taking a good quality fish oil.
-Using coconut oil.
-Eating half a banana before bed.
-Getting out in 1 hour of daylight a day to raise serotonin levels.

06: Other reasons to detox

Processed foods
Processed foods are packed full of toxins which are stored in the fat cells to keep them away from the important organs in the body, and hold no nutritional value.

MSG in foods
Monosodium glutamate, or MSG, is a flavour enhancer found in many foods, especially crisps. It over stimulates the glutamate receptors of the brain, heightening the flavour of the food, making that food addictive.

Glutamic acid is an amino acid that occurs naturally in some foodstuffs. Glutamic acid is known as an excitotoxin. High levels of excitotoxins have been shown in studies on rats to cause damage to areas of the brain, and humans are 5-6 times more sensitive!

Excitotoxins are substances that over excite brain and nerve cells until they die. This then leads to symptoms of migraines, lethargy, ADHD, ADD, cardiac arrhythmia, dizziness, depression, rapid heartbeat and more.

Aspartame
Sweetener found in sweets, chewing gum and many foods.

Aspartame is also an excitotoxin, which stimulates the production of free radicals, which can lead to cancer.

It can also cause serotonin (the happy hormone) to be decreased; this in turn can lead to depression.

Flavours and colouring

Many foods have artificial flavourings and colourings; some are natural – the ones that are not are E 100-199 and E600-699 plus sodium nitrite and MSG E 621. Many of these Es cause cancers, and chronic allergic reactions. Eat organic as much as you can and do not eat anything with artificial additives.

Cooking methods

* **The healthiest cooking vessels to cook with (i.e: sauce pans etc.) are stainless steel, glass and ceramic.**
* **The ones to avoid are aluminium and Teflon coated.**
* **The best cooking methods are steaming, grilling, stir frying and dehydrating.**
* **The worst cooking methods are microwaving, barbecuing and frying on high heat.**

07: Bath products

Part of a good detox is to have a look at the products you use on your body and your home.
If you are about to do a pure detox, you don't want to put toxins back onto your skin for your pores to soak up into your body again!

You can now get chemical free make up everywhere, so buy it! Seriously, it's so much better for you. I use Bare Essential minerals and I also like Liz Earl.

Also look at creams, bath products, what you wash your clothes in, what you clean your dishes in, what you brush your teeth in ... everything! Even paint – you can get chemical free paint, I painted my daughter's bedroom in it, it was called Alvor.

The main product you don't want on your skin is sodium laurel sulphate (SLS). It's potentially harmful to skin and hair, because it cleans by corrosion. If you use SLS you cannot effectively moisturise and it also dries skin by stripping the protective lipids from the surface. And guess what – it's in everything! I bet if you look on your bath products (if they are not chemical free) it will be one of the first ingredients!

There is also a connection of SLS with nitrate contamination. SLS can have a reaction to many types of ingredients used in skin products and forms nitrosomines (nitrates). Nitrates are potential cancer-causing carcinogens.

Have a look at your deodorants – most are made with aluminium and chemicals.

There are a lot of healthy choices now at health food shops, or online.
You can use essential oils for perfumes, coconut oil makes a great cleanser and moisturiser, I even put it in my hair for a deep conditioning treatment.

08: Other products

Look at the clothes you wear and opt for bed linen and sports clothes made with bamboo or organic cotton.

Take electrical equipment out of your bedroom for a good night's sleep and make sure your house is well aired.

Avoid recreational drugs

The three most commonly used recreational drugs in the western world are caffeine, tobacco and alcohol. These can have harmful effects, putting a load on your liver, and they take valuable nutrients out of your body, making you more susceptible to acidity which leads to disease. Aim to stop them, or at least cut back. Dandelion tea is a good alternative to coffee and is excellent for liver cleansing.

09: Foods that help a detox

Coconut oil

Coconut oil is one of the best oils to cook with and eat.

It does not become unstable or carcinogenic when cooked at a high temperature, (unlike most other oils).

Coconut oil is a fantastic defence for the human body against diseases, boosting your immune system.

Coconut oil is a saturated fat, but not all saturated fats are alike; the medium chain triglycerides found in coconut milk are not harmful, they will not raise your cholesterol levels and, incredibly, coconut oil has been found to reduce injuries to the arteries. It also raises your metabolic rate, so helps you lose weight.

Vitamin D

I see many mums slathering factor 50 on their kids in a mad panic that they will get skin cancer immediately if they do not, or forcing caps and long sleeves on the moment the temperature is above 18 degrees C. Don't get me wrong, of course it is important to protect yourself and your children from burning, but are we becoming too obsessed with this?

Alarmingly, consultants are seeing an increase in the disease rickets amongst children.

Vitamin D primary function is for bone health, it modulates neuromuscular function, enhances immunity, enhances gut function, reduces inflammation, and has an influence on stopping the self-mutated cells that cause cancer. And helps you lose weight.

So vitamin D is really needed for optimal health, and factor 50 will stop you absorbing this amazing vitamin.

Ten to fifteen minutes of sun exposure a day gives your body a big dose of vitamin D and is the most natural way of gaining your vit D fix – ever wondered why you feel so much better in the summer than the winter? Well, vit D is your answer.

Vitamin D rich foods – eggs (yolks), fish, cod liver oil, fresh fruit and vegetables – you can even put mushrooms in the sun and they will produce Vitamin D, so if you can't sunbathe, your mushrooms can do it for you.

Green vegetables
Green vegetables are a nutrient-dense source of minerals like magnesium, potassium, manganese, calcium, folate and betaine.
Including...

- **Kale**
- **Chard**
- **Lettuce**
- **Parsley**
- **Spinach**
- **Sweet potato leaves**
- **Baby greens**
- **Endive**

Magnesium
Your mitochondria use magnesium to produce the body's energy currency. Eating greens like spinach and chard will give you a good dietary supplement of magnesium.

Potassium
Potassium is responsible for nerve cell function, protein synthesis, muscle growth, and muscle contractions. (If you get cramps you are probably lacking in potassium (or sodium).

Manganese
Manganese aids in the formation of bones.

Calcium
Leafy greens are a fantastic source of calcium, look what cows eat all day!

Folate
Helps prevent heart disease.

Betaine
Betaine also helps maintain liver health and spinach is one of the best vegetable sources of betaine.

Make sure your eating plan is rich in green vegetables.

Chia seed
Chia seed is a super food and is a complete protein with eight essential amino acids.
It is high in anti-oxidants, and contains seven times more vitamin C than oranges, three times more iron than spinach, and two times more potassium than bananas. It is great for healing the digestion, is high in fibre and balances the blood sugar levels.

Have on smoothies, oats or yogurt and buy from your local health food shop.

Omega 3 oils for fat loss

A recent study has shown that taking fish oil supplements, with regular exercise, can
assist weight loss.

Seventy-five overweight and obese people were put into four groups, taking various oils. The study by the University of South Australia showed that the group that were given the fish oil and had done the exercise showed a decrease in body fat percentage plus an average 2kg/4.5lb weight loss.
You can lose up to 2 pounds a month just by taking omega 3 fish oils alone.
If you are a vegetarian, milled flaxseeds are a good source of Omega 3.

Other foods with omega 3 are
- **chia seeds**
- **fish**
- **broccoli**
- **flaxseeds**
- **oil, and walnuts.**

Acid and alkaline foods

Acid and alkaline are found in foods we eat.

An acidic body will decrease the body's ability to absorb vitamins and minerals, damage cells, and make a bad atmosphere for detoxification. Processed foods and a high animal/dairy diet contribute towards an acid environment.

- **To maintain health, the diet should consist of 60% alkaline forming foods and 40% acid forming foods.**

- **To restore health, the diet should consist of 80% alkaline forming foods and 20% acid forming foods.**

Generally, alkaline forming foods include:

most fruits, green vegetables, peas, beans, lentils, spices, herbs and seasonings, and seeds and nuts.

Generally, acid forming foods include:

meat, fish, poultry, eggs, grains, and legumes.

When you do your detox, make sure you eat plenty of fruit and vegetables to allow for a less hostile acidic environment, and alkalise your body.

. . . .

Fermented foods

We have been fermenting food all over the world, since ancient times; evidence has been found in Babylon around 5000 BC, ancient Egypt circa 3150 BC, pre-Hispanic Mexico circa 2000 BC, and Sudan circa 1500 BC.

As we are now living with antibiotic drugs, chlorinated water and antibacterial soap; if we fail to replenish the good bacteria, we won't effectively get nutrients out of the food we're eating.

Fermenting our foods before we eat them is like partially digesting them before we consume them.

Sometimes people who cannot tolerate milk can eat yogurt. This is because the lactose in milk is broken down as the milk is fermented and turns into yogurt.

Fermented foods restore the proper balance of bacteria in the gut.

Bad bacteria in the gut can lead to asthma, lactose intolerance gluten intolerance, constipation, irritable bowel syndrome, yeast infections, allergies – all of these conditions have been linked to a lack of good bacteria in the gut.

Raw, fermented foods are rich in enzymes, and actually increase the vitamin content.

Eating fermented food helps us to absorb the nutrients we're consuming and helps to preserve it for longer periods of time. It can also increase the flavour.

10: Supplements and foods that can help you in a detoxification

- **Spirulina** - great for balancing the blood sugars.
- **Wheatgrass** - contains 100 enzymes, 12 vitamins and 21 amino acids – great in smoothies/juices.
- **Linseeds/milled flaxseeds.**
- **Acidopholis** - good bacteria for the gut.
- **Psyllium husks** - very fibrous and fills you up.
- **Spa-tone sports** - is an amazing liquid iron supplement that will boost your energy.

11: Foods to avoid to cut belly fat

Packaged foods, partially hydrogenated oils, enriched flours and trans fats.

Researchers have found that the trans fats, found in margarine, packaged biscuits, crackers and pasta, increase fat in your midsection, and can actually redistribute fat from other parts of the body to the belly.

Foods that fight belly fat
Eat more monounsaturated fats, found in nuts, olive oil and seeds;
also include avocados, and whole grains.

12: Sleep

It always amazes me how little sleep my clients get before they start with me, and they wonder why they feel so low in energy?
Whenever they do my detox plan, their sleep patterns dramatically change. This is because we eliminate high levels of caffeine, sugar, stress, alcohol and these are all the reasons you can be either unable to get to sleep, have broken sleep or wake up too early.
Other reasons are your poor digestion could be keeping you awake or in a shallow sleep, and your poor nutrient levels could be stopping you getting a night of slumber.

Other ways I suggest my clients aid their sleep is having no electrical devices in the bedroom.
So no phones, TVs, computers, etc.I If your phone and computer are in the bedroom, chances are you will be doing work on them – yes? Emails etc. So then you are not associating your gorgeous and tranquil bed with beautiful slumber, you will associate that room with stress. Again, create the mood, the subliminal messages in your life – this is your life, your advert, you create it!

Reasons lack of sleep leads to you being FAT!
High cortisol levels attribute to fat gain and this delightful hormone will be high if you don't sleep.
You will also have more lethargy, so you are less likely to exercise well.
You are likely to eat more because your blood sugar levels will not be balanced.
So sleep – eight hours a night.

13: Water

You may not know this, but if you do not drink enough water you will gain weight!
Being dehydrated makes you FAT! Why?

- **Because you are likely to eat more if you are dehydrated.**

- **Because the amount of calories you burn a day is controlled by your liver (metabolism) and if your kidneys are dehydrated, your liver won't function efficiently.**

- **You can get water retention if you don't drink enough, which can make you look swollen.**

- **Drinking water before a meal fills you up.**

Have 2 litres a day.

During your detox your skin, hair, nails and eyes all become bright and younger looking. Your posture will improve, which instantly makes you look younger; your stomach will get a lot flatter, and we always associate small waistlines with youth; your flexibility will massively improve, which means you will walk with agility, and you will be bouncing off the walls with energy!

I can't wait to help you to get there!

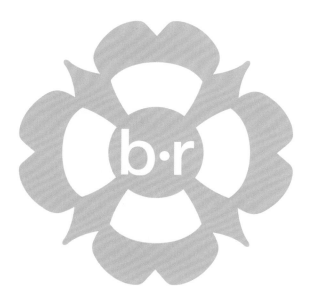

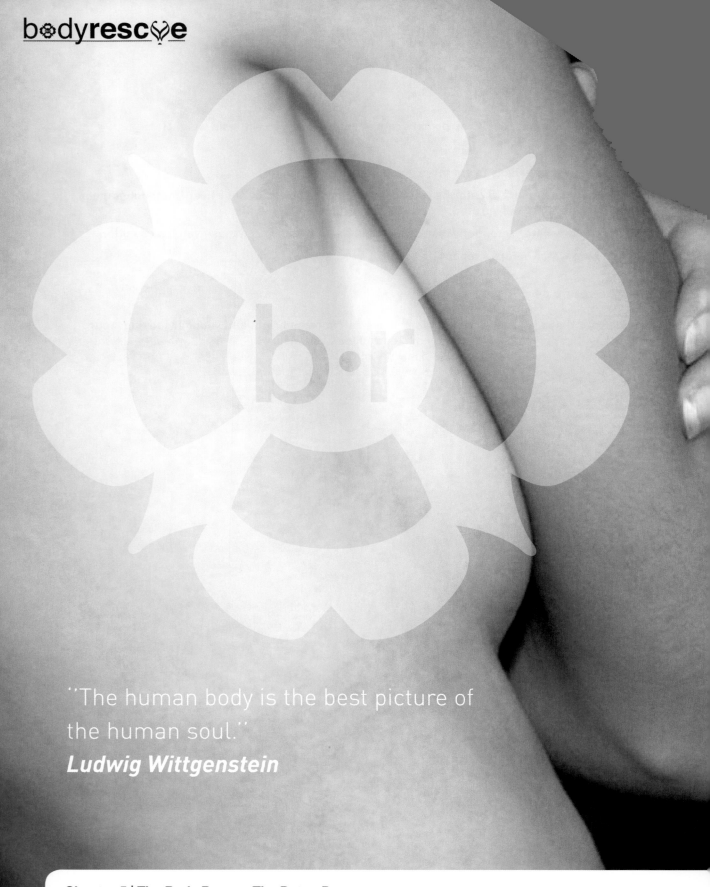

bodyrescue

''The human body is the best picture of the human soul.''
Ludwig Wittgenstein

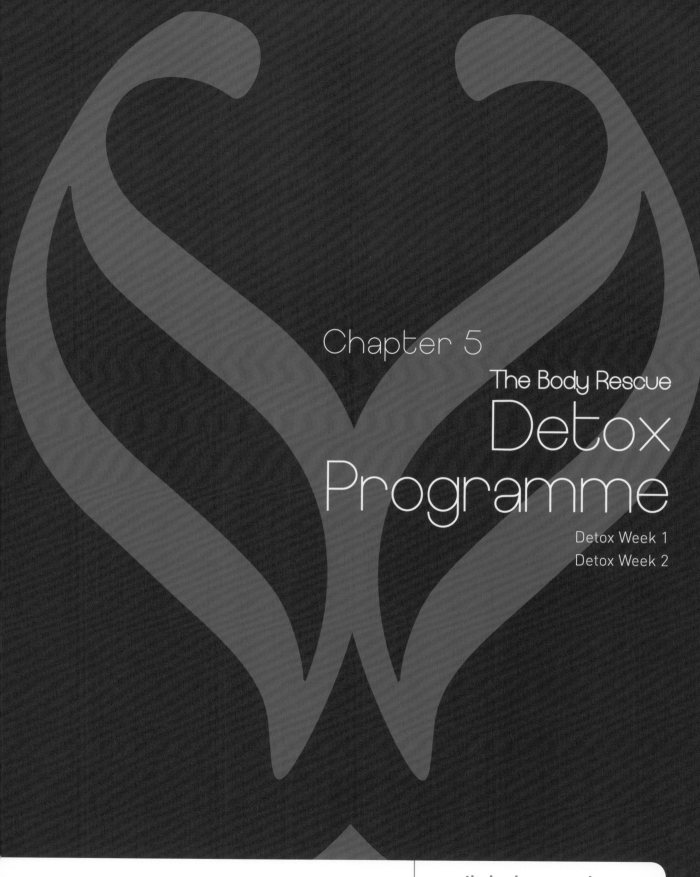

Chapter 5

The Body Rescue
Detox
Programme

Detox Week 1
Detox Week 2

....

Please note the detox programme is not suitable for pregnant or breastfeeding women.
If you have any doubts about your health please contact your Dr prior to starting
The Body Rescue Plan.

....

My detox programme is really simple, and you will not go hungry.
The only symptom you may have is headaches from cutting out caffeine, but the fact that that caffeine gives you a headache is a huge indicator as to why you do not need it in your life! You may also have a few days of craving sugar/carbs, but this will not last any longer than 5 days max, usually only 2-3 days. So 2-3 days is worth a lifetime of feeling amazing, right?

I recently read a magazine article on the best feelings you get in the world. One of the top one hundred feelings was day four of a detox!

You will feel so amazing after three days, and you may even feel amazing from day one.
Just being in control of your foods and energy levels is really empowering. Some people find they react strongly to their abstinence from tea and coffee, usually getting headaches. Its highly likely after three days the headaches will go, so stick with it – and look, if you get such strong headaches from giving up a so called food, what on earth is it doing to your poor body?

I know we are a nation of tea and coffee drinkers, and it all seems like the norm, but from my professional opinion and observation, I would say we are a nation of addicts with no real energy, and this is mainly due to our caffeine obsession.
During your detox you may also feel irritable, your skin may react when the toxins come out, or you may get flu-like symptoms. It really depends how many toxins are in there, but the stronger the reaction the more you must be resilient to the fight against those toxins. Get them out of you and start living!

Here it is...

Detox week 1-2

Week 1

- **Eat as much white meat as you want.**
  (If you are vegetarian you may have pulses instead of meat.)
- **Eat as much fish as you want**
  (including shellfish). High levels of mercury are in swordfish, tilefish and shark,
  so best to avoid these.
- **Eat as much vegetables, sprouted foods and fruit as you want**
  (except bananas).
- **Eat herbs and spices.**
- **Have one fistful of nuts and seeds and one fistful of dried fruit a day.** (Milled flaxseeds are amazing.) (N.B. Fistful, not handful.)
- **Eggs are allowed.**
- **Vinegar.** (Nothing else added.)
- **Eat more vegetables than fruit, but eat as much fruit as you like.**

TOP TIP
- **Apple cider vinegar is particularly good for detoxing,**
  it is full of minerals and vitamins and enzymes and is amazing for the immune system.
- **Herbal teas and coconut water are good.**
- **You can also have corn, sweet potato and other root vegetables,**
  except no white potato.
- **Drinks** – herbal teas, coconut water, water, fresh juices.

That's it, nothing else
- No dairy, alcohol, carbs, sugar, red meat, caffeine or anything packaged.
- 2-3 litres of water a day.

TOP TIP
- **If you have a sweet tooth go and buy some Nakd bars,** you are allowed all the flavours from week 1 except cocoa, which you are allowed from week 3. They are really delicious. BUT, make sure you allow for this with the allocated one fistful of nuts/seeds and one fistful of dried fruit. One Nakd bar is about half a fistful of both nuts, seeds and dried fruit, so two Nakd bars would be your daily quota.

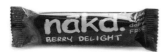

  Do not use the Nakd bars with added oats or soya for the detox.
- **Almond and cashew spread are also really yummy.**
- **I also find liquorice tea really good for calming my sweet tooth.**

TOP TIP
- **Dried nori strips (seaweed) are a delicious snack and really nutritious,**
  eat as much as you like – a great crisp alternative.

Week 2

- **Same as week 1,**
  but add one fistful of carbs a day in oats, couscous, brown rice, wholemeal pasta, potatoes, buckwheat, amaranth and quinoa– once a week go wheat free. (If you are sensitive to insulin spikes, avoid potatoes this week.)

- **Plus two tablespoons of coconut oil or one tablespoon of olive oil.**

- **You may have olives, but count them as part of your olive oil quota,**
  so ten olives is one tablespoon of olive oil.

- **You may have coconut slices dried, but have this as part of your dried fruit quota,**
  and no added anything.

- **Natural yogurt.**
  (If you do not eat dairy, try other yogurts, but no added nasties.)

- **Bananas**

TOP TIP

I would really advise that you take spirulina, and or psyllium husks, thirty minutes before you eat in the morning and thirty minutes before your afternoon snack. It will help with your digestion, fill you up and balance your blood sugar levels, so you are not tempted to eat out of tiredness. You can find these in health food shops.

Juicing

To help aid a detox it is a really good idea to juice some of your fruit and vegetables. You can use a blender for making fruit smoothies or a vegetable juicer for vegetables and hard fruits like apples. Or, if you want an all singing, all dancing vegetable and fruit juicer, that doesn't chuck out the pulp and can also make soups, I would recommend Vitamix. www.vitamix.com

Benefits of juicing

-The nutrients are easily absorbed.
-They have high antioxidants and phytochemicals, which are protective against cellular damage.
-Green juices are high in chlorophyll, which is good for your red blood cells, and green vegetables aid weight loss.
-Red, purple and blue juices reduce inflammation in the body.
-Adding the cruciferous vegetable group to smoothies can aid weight loss.

Cruciferous vegetables

- **Cauliflower** (white or purple)
- **Broccoli** (green or purple)
- **Brussels sprouts**
- **Kale** (green or purple)
- **Bok choy** (chinese cabbage or pak choi)
- **Cabbage** (green, red or purple)
- **Collard greens**
- **Watercress**
- **Radish**
- **Broccoli sprouts**
- **Rocket**
- **Mustard greens**
- **Turnip**

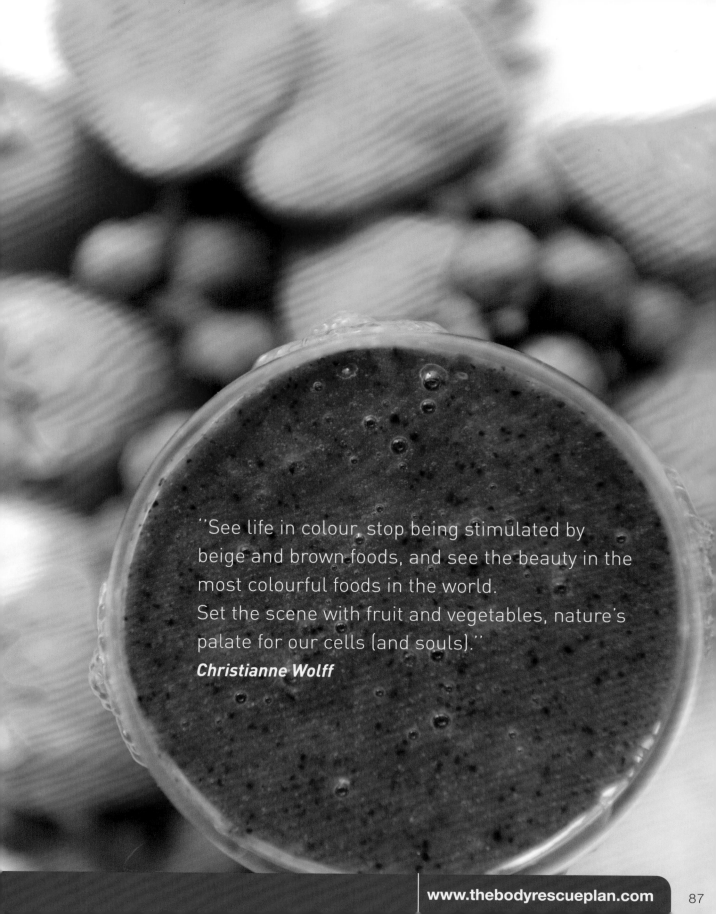

"See life in colour, stop being stimulated by beige and brown foods, and see the beauty in the most colourful foods in the world.
Set the scene with fruit and vegetables, nature's palate for our cells (and souls)."
Christianne Wolff

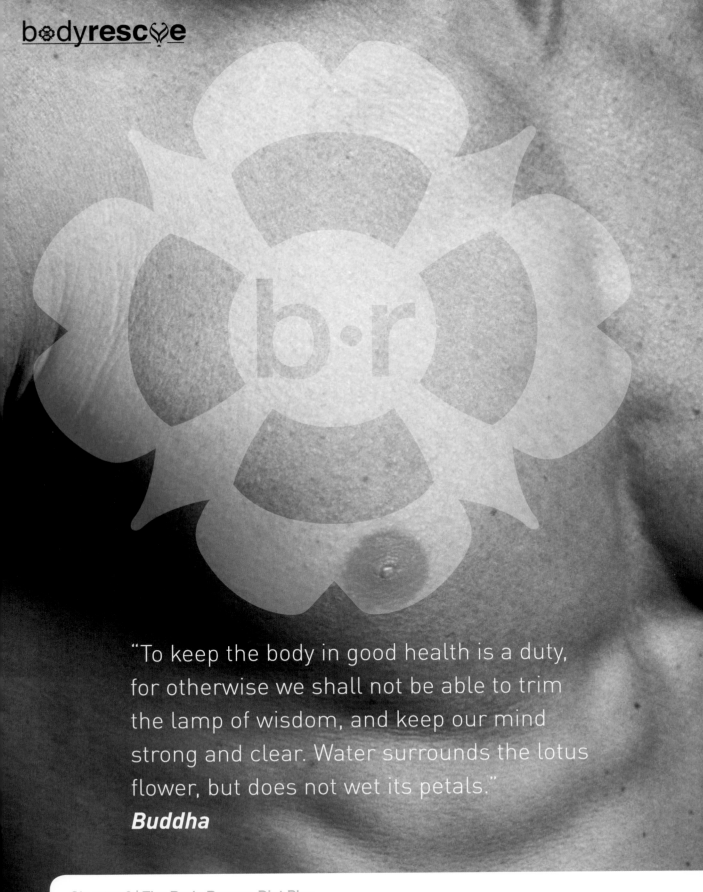

bodyrescue

"To keep the body in good health is a duty, for otherwise we shall not be able to trim the lamp of wisdom, and keep our mind strong and clear. Water surrounds the lotus flower, but does not wet its petals."
Buddha

Chapter 6

The Body Rescue
Diet Plan

Weeks 3-12 eating plan
(after the Detox Plan)

01: Get organised

02: Creating associations

03: A note about breakfast

04: Weeks 1-12 eating plan

05: Maintenance

After the 2 week detox you are now ready to go onto my Body Rescue diet plan. This is just 10 weeks of re-introducing foods into your system and savouring the textures, tastes, and smells.

01: Get organised

The key to sticking to any programme that is different to your routine already, is to get organised!

Write in your diary
(example diary in Chapter 10) where you will fit the exercise in and plan it like it is a meeting.

Plan out your week's food in advance,
and what meals you will have, so that you are really excited to eat them.

Eat organic.
I know it is more expensive, but if you are detoxing, your body will love you for living off chemical free food! I would really recommend Abel and Cole, they are a home delivery organic service and are much cheaper than your average supermarket selling organic foods. They also have wonderful cookbooks and a great ethos! If you are strapped for cash, use your local farm shop or market and buy an abundance of fresh fruit, veg, and fish for probably half the price of a supermarket, if not less.

02: Creating associations

The moment people go on a diet they often seem to somehow switch off the creative part of their brain. I've seen people eat a diet of Broccoli and salmon every day in a bid to get slim, with no effort and celebration in the foods they are eating.

When you eat, how are you eating?
Are you chewing enough?
You need to chew 33 times, please – this not only allows mastication to break down the foods so you can digest them as best as possible, it also gives you time to realise you are full and appreciate the wonderful foods you are eating.

Do you eat whilst walking?

Do you eat whilst on the computer, phone, TV, on a train, at work?

What do you use to eat out of?

Are you eating out of plastic packaging, with a plastic fork or spoon?

Do you eat at a table?

How long do you spend eating?

Do you have a house full of junk food?

What is your association with lots of packaged foods?

What is your association with colourful fruits and vegetables?

This is your life and you are setting the scene, so make it a good one.
Imagine you are having a fine dining experience, would you wharf through every mouthful, or would you slowly appreciate and savour each mouthful. If you buy food out of plastic you will have a totally different appreciation and experience with your foods.

When you look at food adverts they sex up the foods, the colours are bright, the people who eat them are beautifully dressed, they lure you in, the lighting would be dimly lit.

So why not create that scene for yourself. Why not create your own advert that has subliminal messages?

- **Use crockery you love, it doesn't have to be posh, but you should enjoy eating from it.**
- **Create colour in your food, so it touches your senses.**
- **Use amazing smells (i.e. use herbs, spices, and anything that smells good).**
- **Use many textures in your foods to fulfil your senses.**
- **Listen to music that slows you down and chills you out, whilst eating.**
- **Enjoy the preparation of food, put love into it, remember the energy you put into it, you will be absorbing.**
- **Chew your food!**
- **Take your time**

Have a clean kitchen that is abundant with colour in fresh foods.

-This then becomes your new association, you may have been programmed into salivating each time you see an advert for chocolate or Coke, now it's time to re-programme, so that you adore what you eat and all your surroundings, you feel like you have come home!

You do not have to be a great cook to prepare foods and it certainly does not have to take hours of your time. I am not a natural at cooking, but I create a scene in the kitchen that is fun and vibrant and makes me feel good. I will not spend more than thirty minutes on any meal!

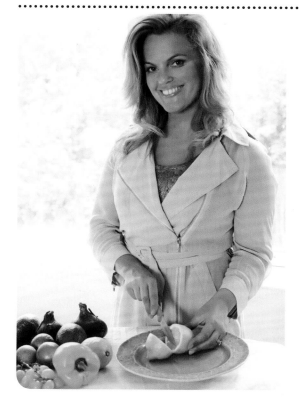

03: A note about breakfast

Please never skip breakfast, it is a very important meal of the day and will balance your blood sugars, so you do not get the mid-morning munchies – as well as that if you eat in the morning it sends a trigger to your metabolism to burn fat for the day, if you skip breakfast your metabolic rate will lower as your body will think it's starving and hold onto fat.

It is a good idea to try and get some protein for breakfast, or even have a full protein breakfast on some days – there have been many studies researched on the effect of having protein for breakfast, which shows evidence of people feeling fuller for longer. Protein in general will give you a fuller feeling than carbs, with less calories than carbs.

04: Weeks 3-12 Eating plan (after the Detox Plan)

(Detox plan week 1 and 2) and then...

Week 3
Same as week 2 of the detox plus you may add...
One matchbox size piece of cheese, or two matchbox size pieces of goats' cheese a day.
As much pulses as you like (lentils, beans, chickpeas etc.) add soy if you are vegetarian.
One tablespoon of carob or cocoa a day. (You can have cocoa Nakd bars this week.)
Vanilla essence (1tsp) in cooking.
2.5 litres of water.

Week 4
Same as above, plus you may now also add...
One tablespoon a day of either Xylitol, Stevia, honey, maple syrup, Yacon, date sugar, coconut sugar, agave nectar. These are natural sweeteners. Never use artificial sweeteners.
Plus one fistful of buckwheat, polenta, coconut flour or rice flour a week (yummy for making pancakes and baking).

Week 5
Same as above, plus you may have...
1 tablespoon of Cornflour a week.
One glass of coconut milk a day.
Soya sauce.

Week 6
Same as above, plus you may have...
One glass of rice milk or almond milk a day.

One handful of red meat a week.

Week 7
Same as above, plus you may have...
One alcoholic spirit or one small glass organic wine. (One for the week- this is not a necessity.)

Week 8
The same as above

Week 9
The same as above

Weeks 10 and 11
Will be the 2 week detox again- please prepare!

Week 12
Same as week 5

05: Maintenance

If you have now reached your goal weight and are happy with the way you look and feel, then eat clean in the week as week 6 and allow one cheat day at the weekend (or whatever suits your schedule). Some people feel they can have two cheat days a week, but monitor how you look and feel for that. Remember, if you are very addicted to sugar, caffeine or alcohol, it may be very difficult for you to just have it for one or two days, and perhaps is better cut out for a little longer or forever. There are plenty of delicious sweet foods that don't have to have sugar in, and it's your call on caffeine or alcohol. What you have to ask yourself is, do I feel in control or is it controlling me?

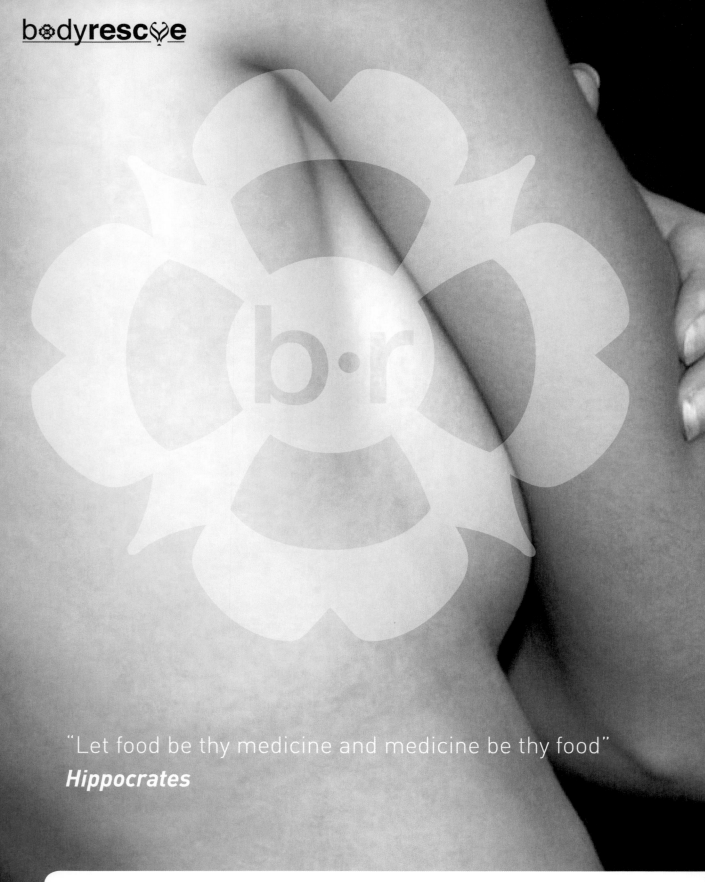

"Let food be thy medicine and medicine be thy food"
Hippocrates

Chapter 7
Recipes and shopping list

01: Breakfast recipes 1
02: Smoothies & Juices
03: Breakfast recipes 2
04: Lunch and Supper recipes
05: Yummy snacks and puddings
06: Body Rescue Diet Plan
07: 7 day Body Rescue Diet Plan recipes
08: Shopping list

Here are some delicious recipes for you to enjoy; please make sure you eat them on the right days. The days you are meant to eat them are written beside them for your convenience.

01: Breakfast

Week 1 onwards
Breakfast ideas...

- Boiled eggs and asparagus soldiers
- Poached eggs and salmon
- Omelette
- Kippers
- Fruit salad

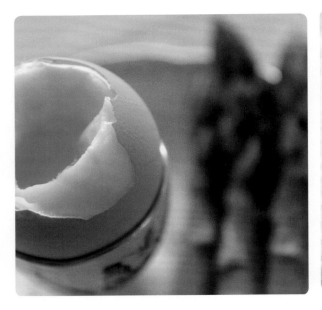
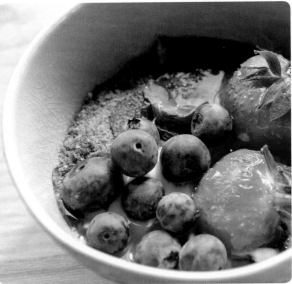

02: Smoothies & Juices

Smoothies are made with a blender.

Juices are made with a vegetable juicer, I would thoroughly recommend Vitamix.

Vegetable juices...

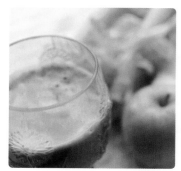

Kale and apple surprise juice
Serves 1
2 green apples
1 Bunch of kale
3 celery stalks
1 cucumber
½ lemon
1 (1 inch) piece fresh ginger
Process these through a vegetable juicer and enjoy.

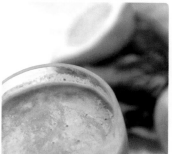

Carrot and spinach
Serves 1
3 large carrots
½ lemon
1 bunch of Spinach leaves
1 apple
Process these through a vegetable juicer and enjoy.

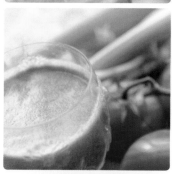

Tomato juice
Serves 1
1 handfull of tomatoes
1 stalk celery
1 cucumber
½ teaspoon (tsp) Himalaya sea salt; pepper; cayenne pepper
Process these through a vegetable juicer and enjoy.

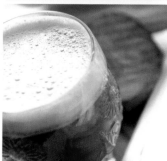

Immune booster
Serves 1
1 beetroot
3 large carrots
4 stalks celery
½ cucumber
½ thumb of ginger
1 medium pear
Process these through a vegetable juicer and enjoy.

Smoothies in...
1. Mango and pineapple
2. Strawberries and mango
3. Strawberries and blueberries

 1 2 3

Just put the ingredients in a blender until smooth. Add ice if you want. Add milled flaxseeds as a topping to thicken up

Smoothies

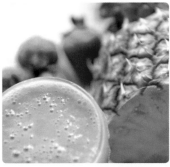
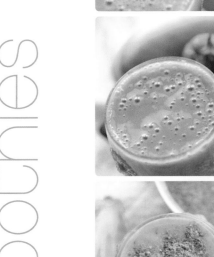
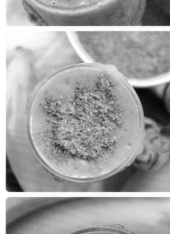

Week 2 till 9 and 10 -12
Strawberry & banana smoothie
Serves 1
¼ pineapple
6 strawberries
½ banana
1 glass of water
1 tsp flax seed oil

Just put the ingredients in a blender until smooth. Add ice if you want. Add milled flaxseeds as a topping to thicken up.

Week 2 till 9 and 10-12
Tropicana body smoothie
Serves 1
1 banana, frozen
4 strawberries
1 glass of water
1 tsp flax oil (optional)

Just put the ingredients in a blender until smooth. Add ice if you want. Add milled flaxseeds as a topping to thicken up.

Week 2 till 9 and 10-12
Red mango and banana surprise smoothie
Serves 1
½ mango
¼ tsp natural coconut oil
4 strawberries, frozen
½ banana, frozen
1 glass of water
1 tsp flax oil (optional)

Week 2 till 9 and 10-12
Banana and berry smoothie
Serves 1
½ pear
10 blueberries or frozen mixed berries
½ banana, frozen
1 glass of water
1 pinch of cinnamon

Just put the ingredients in a blender until smooth. Add ice if you want. Add milled flaxseeds as a topping to thicken up.

03: Breakfast

Week 5 till 9, 12

High protein pancakes

Sugar and wheat FREE pancakes, add agave nectar if you wish.
Serves 4 pancakes.

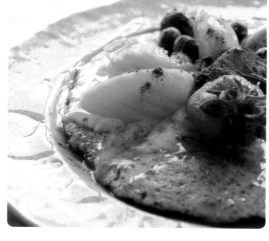

Ingredients

240g ground almonds
¼ tablespoon (tbsp) milled flaxseed.
¼ tsp baking soda.
1 large egg
60g unsweetened almond milk.
240g coconut milk.
2 tbsp's coconut oil, melted.

Preparation method

1 Mix the ground almonds, flaxseed, and baking soda.
2 In a separate bowl, whisk the eggs, then add the milk and oil and whisk together.
3 Whisk the mixtures together, gradually and add more milk if needed, one tablespoon at a time, to make a nice pancake batter.
4 Lightly oil a frying pan and heat over medium heat, and pour ¼ cup batter into it.
5 Cook for three mins each side.
6 Serve with fruit, agave nectar, Greek yogurt etc.

Makes 4-6 four-inch pancakes.

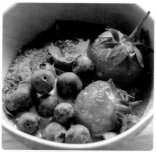

Weeks 4 to 8, and 11-12

Fruit, yogurt and flaxseeds

Yogurt, milled flaxseed and agave nectar with some berries makes a delicious snack or breakfast.

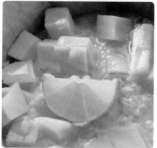

Weeks 5 till 9, 11,12

Mango, lime and coconut porridge

Porridge oats cooked in coconut milk, lime, mango and agave nectar is truly scrumptious.

Lunch and
Supper recipes

Weeks 1 till 12 if used without oil

Salad Niçoise

Serves 1

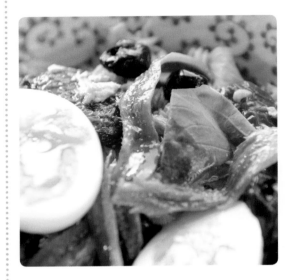

Ingredients

1 egg
100 grams sun blush tomatoes in oil
1 tin of tuna
Lettuce leaves
2 tsp extra virgin olive oil
Juice of ½ lemon
Pinch of salt
4 anchovy fillets
1 handful fresh basil leaves

Preparation method

1 Boil egg for 5 mins.

2 Whisk lemon juice, oil and salt and pour over all the ingredients for a delicious salad (you could use this in week 1 without the oil).

04:

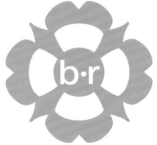

Week 2 till 9, then 10-12
Courgette noodles
Makes a yummy alternative to any noodle dish
Serves 2

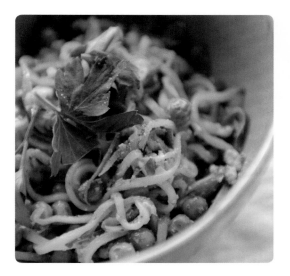

Ingredients
2 good sized courgettes

Sauce
1 tsp coconut oil
3 cloves of garlic, chopped finely
1 large bunch of basil leaves
1 cup of lightly toasted pine nuts
4 tbsp of fresh or frozen peas
salt and pepper
lemon zest and Parmesan cheese, to finish

Preparation method
1 Grate the courgette in long strokes along a julienne grater.

2 Make the pesto sauce by placing the basil leaves, pine nuts and 1 garlic clove in to a blender.

4 Gently fry the courgette with the garlic, then stir in the pesto and the frozen peas.

4 Stir until coated, season with salt and pepper, then take off the heat.

5 Serve on a bed of green leaves. (For a week 3 version add grated cheese)

Weeks 2 to 8, 10 and 11,12
Courgettes and almonds
Serves 4

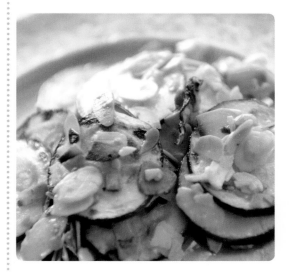

Ingredients
2 tbsp coconut oil
2 tbsp flaked almonds
350g courgette finely sliced

Preparation method
1 Heat coconut oil in a pan and add the almonds for 2 mins, stirring.

2 Add courgette and toss with the oil and almonds until cooked, season to taste and serve with a fish dish or as a nice snack.

This makes a really meaty meal out of a courgette.

Weeks 2 till 9, 10 and 11,12

Egg fried rice
Serves 2

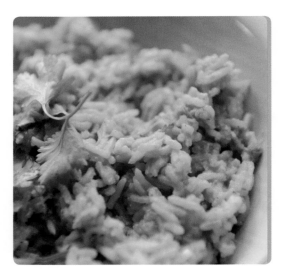

Ingredients
4fl oz (125ml) basmati rice
1 large egg, beaten, 2 spring onions
Pinch of salt
1 tbsp oil
1tbsp soy sauce

Preparation method
1 Cook the rice for 15 mins in a pan with a lid, on a low heat, without stirring or lifting the lid.

2 Allow the rice to go cold and fluff it up with a fork.

3 Fry the onions with half the oil for 3 mins. Add lemon juice and pepper

4 Next add the rest of the oil to the pan with the rice and cook for 30 seconds.

5 Continue to spread the ingredients around the pan and add the beaten egg.

6 Finally, add the spring onion and soy sauce.

To bulk this out I love adding shiitake mushrooms or green vegetables, with tuna fish.

Week 3 onward, if not using soy sauce.

If using soy sauce week 5 till 9...

...and then 10,11,12

Prawn stir fry noodles
Serves 2

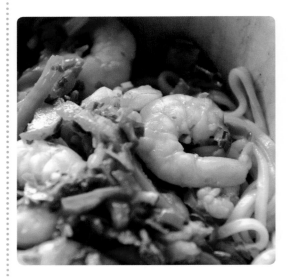

Ingredients
200g raw, peeled tiger prawns
1 chilli, chopped, 2-3 garlic cloves crushed,
1 bunch coriander, 1 lime- juice,
3 tbsp fish sauce (make sure there is no added sugar), 2 tbsp coconut oil, Small piece ginger, finely sliced, 8 spring onions, finely sliced
1 red pepper, thinly sliced 150g bean sprouts
1 tbsp soy sauce

Noodles and lime wedges to serve.

Preparation method
1 Put the chilli, crushed garlic and coriander in a blender. Add half of the lime juice and the fish sauce, then pour this over the prawns in a bowl.

2 Heat 1 tbsp of coconut oil in a wok and add the ginger and spring onions and fry for 1 min. Add the red pepper and fry for a further minute. Add the bean sprouts and fry for another 2 mins. Add the soy sauce if on week 5.

3 Fry the prawns for 2 mins and add the marinade, then pour onto the vegetable dish.

4 Serve with noodles and sprinkle with coriander.

Weeks 3-8 and 11,12
Lentil shepherd's pie
Serves 4

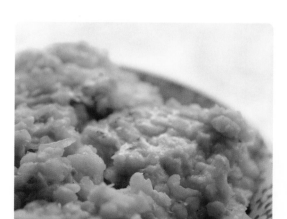

Ingredients
1 tbsp coconut oil, 1 large onion, halved and sliced, 2 large carrots cut into small cubes, 2 tbsp thyme chopped, 400g can chopped tomatoes, 2 vegetable stock cubes, 270g red lentils, 1000g sweet potatoes, peeled and cut into chunks, 25g coconut oil, 100g mature cheddar, grated

Preparation method
1 Heat the oil in a frying pan, then fry the onion until golden. Add the carrots, 150ml water and the tomatoes, then add in the stock cubes and simmer for 10 mins. Wash the lentils and add; cook until the carrots still have a bit of bite and the lentils are pulpy.

2 Meanwhile, boil the sweet potatoes for 15 mins. and then mash with the coconut oil. Place the lentil and vegetable mix in an ovenproof dish and layer the sweet potato on top. Sprinkle the cheese and thyme on top of that and cook in the oven at 190°C/170°C fan/gas 5. Cook for 20 mins until golden and hot all the way through.

Serve with mixed vegetables of your choice.

Weeks 3-8 and 11, 12
Lentil curry
Serves 4

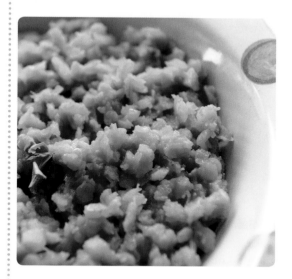

Ingredients
200g (8oz) red lentils, ½ large onion, diced, ½ tbsp coconut oil, ½ tbsp curry paste, ½ tbsp curry powder, ½ tbsp ground turmeric, ½ tbsp ground cumin, ½ tbsp chilli powder, ½ tbsp salt, ½ tbsp garlic, ½ tbsp ginger root minced, 1 can tomato puree

Preparation method
1 Wash the lentils and boil in a pan.

2 Meanwhile caramelise the onions in the coconut oil.

3 Place the curry paste, curry powder, turmeric, cumin, chilli powder, salt, garlic, and ginger in a mixing bowl, and mix. Add the curry mixture to the caramelised onions and cook over a high heat stirring constantly for 1 to 2 mins.

4 Stir in the tomato puree and reduce heat; allow the curry base to simmer until the lentils are ready.

5 When the lentils are ready drain and mix the curry paste into the lentils and serve immediately.

6 Add rice to serve or eat on its own.

Weeks 3-8 and 11,12
Feta cheese salad

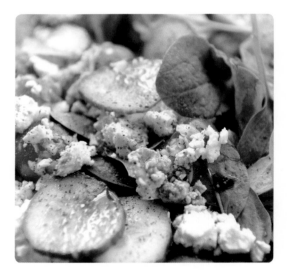

Ingredients and method
Combine all the following ingredients for a quick, easy and delicious fresh salad:
fresh spinach
tomatoes (chopped)
cucumbers (sliced)
red onion (sliced)
spring onion
red pepper (chopped)
feta cheese
olive oil
balsamic vinegar
ground black pepper

Weeks 3-8 and 11,12
Jacket potato and salad

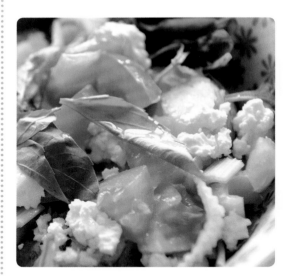

Ingredients
spinach
mixed veggies
2 tbsp's of feta cheese
1 jacket potato
coconut oil

Weeks 4-8 and week 12
Ingredients
Hummus with carrots and cucumber.

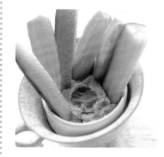

Week 3-8, 11, 12
Stuffed butternut squash
Serves 4

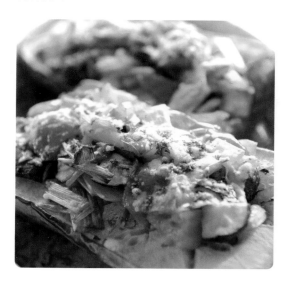

Ingredients
2 medium-sized butternut squash, 2 garlic cloves, peeled and crushed, 1 lemon juiced, dried red chilli flakes, 1 tsp fresh thyme leaves, 1 courgette, 2 leeks, salt and freshly ground black pepper, 200g cherry tomatoes, 2 tbsp finely chopped fresh flat-leaf parsley, 2 level tbsp grated Parmesan cheese, 1 tbsp olive oil (could be used in week 1 without the cheese)

Preparation method
1 Preheat the oven to 200°C/Gas 6.

2 Cut the squash in half, scoop out the seeds then cut criss-cross patterns into the flesh of each one.

3 Mix together the garlic, lemon juice, chilli flakes and thyme and brush this mixture over the flesh.

4 Place the squash in a baking dish, cut side up, and bake in the oven for about 30-40 mins or until the flesh is tender.

5 Meanwhile put the courgette, red pepper and leeks in a separate baking dish and cover with some oil. Season and bake for about 20-25 mins until tender.

6 Add the cherry tomatoes and cook for another 10 mins.

7 Mix the parsley and grated Parmesan together.

8 Arrange the roasted vegetables in the squash halves and put the cheese mix on top to bake for 10 mins. and serve. Gorgeous!

Week 4 till 9, 12
Butternut squash and couscous salad
Serves 2

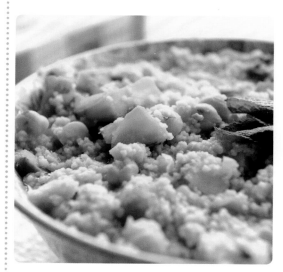

Ingredients
½ butternut squash, ½ tsp coconut oil, ½ small red onion finely chopped, 1 garlic cloves peeled and crushed, ½ tsp cumin seeds, ½ tsp ground coriander, ½ can chickpeas drained, 80g couscous, vegetable stock, 1 tbsp finely chopped coriander

Preparation method
1 Preheat oven to 200°C/180C, fan/gas 6. Put the squash in the oven for 15-20 mins until soft.

2 While the squash is roasting, add hot water to the couscous to cook. Heat the coconut oil in a pan and add the onion and cook for 2-3 mins. Add the garlic, cumin and ground coriander and cook for 2 mins. Remove from the heat. Add the chickpeas and couscous- stir in the fresh coriander.

3 To serve add a fresh salad of small tomatoes, mint and spinach leaves.

Week 4 till 9, 12
Buckwheat pizza
Serves 2

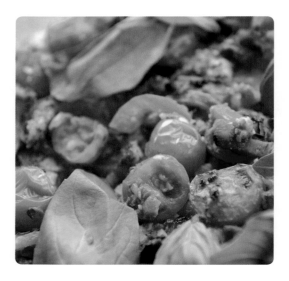

(Buckwheat is not wheat and is gluten free, it is derived from a seed of a flowering plant and has many health benefits, it also strengthens capillary walls because it contains rutin.)

Ingredients
Pizza
60g chia seeds, 1 glass water, 3 tbsp whole grain buckwheat flour, 1 tsp dried oregano, 1 tbsp chopped pine nuts, 1 tbsp chopped pumpkin seeds, 1 tbsp chopped sunflower seeds, 1 tsp sea salt

Topping
60g tomato paste, 12 cherry tomatoes, halved, 3 sliced mushrooms, ½ red pepper, fresh basil leaves, 1-2 tsp dried oregano, 2 spring onions, ½ red onion, salt & pepper to taste, 1 oz goats cheddar cheese, grated

Preparation method
1 Mix the chia seeds, water, buckwheat flour, oregano & salt until the mixture starts to thicken up. **2** Add chopped seeds and nuts. **3** Form the dough into a pizza base on parchment paper and flatten to about 1 cm for a firm thin crust.
4 Bake at 175°C (350°F) for 30-40 mins.
5 Remove from the oven and add the Topping (or make your own topping) and place back in the oven for 10 mins.

A delicious low grain pizza!

Weeks 5 – 8, 12
Tamari salmon noodles
Serves 4

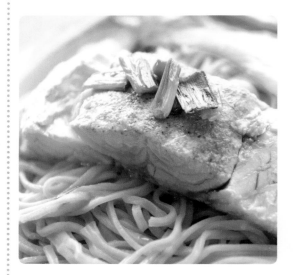

Ingredients
4 salmon fillets, skinless & boneless
4 tsp tamari sauce
2 tsp fresh chilli
4 pak choi leaves

4 servings of dried noodles

Serve with stir fry vegetables.

Preparation method
1 Preheat the oven to 200°C/Gas 6. Place Tamari sauce on each salmon fillet, with the chilli.

2 Place the salmon on top of the pak choi and wrap, place in the oven and cook for around 15 mins.

3 Meanwhile stir fry your vegetables, and keep warm.

4 Cook the noodles.

5 Remove the salmon and place on top of the noodles to serve immediately with the stir-fry vegetables on the side.

I like to add miso soup paste or vegetable stock to have a soup consistency, which is really filling.

Week 6,7,8,12.

Spiced coconut prawns
Serves 1

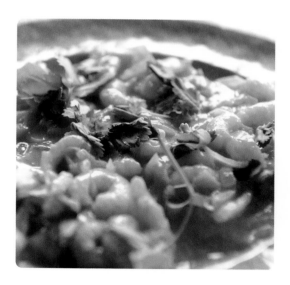

Ingredients
1 tsp rapeseed oil
80g finely chopped onion
1 finely chopped garlic
1 tsp ground cumin
1 tsp ground coriander
½ tsp curry powder
125ml coconut milk
100g peeled jumbo prawns
1 tsp corn flour
1 tbsp water
2 tbsp chopped fresh coriander

Preparation method
1 Sauté onion and garlic for 3 mins, add cumin, coriander and curry powder and cook for 1 min. Stir in coconut milk. Bring to the boil and then simmer for 2 mins.

2 Stir in prawns and cook for about 4 mins, check prawns are ready.

3 Add cornflour mixed in a tablespoon of water to the prawn mixture, and cook until sauce is thicker.

4 Add coriander and serve.

Other creative delicious ideas..

- Millet cauliflower
- Roasted vegetables
- Fish cakes with sweet potatoes
- Pumpkin soup
- Quinoa falafels
- Asian vegetable noodle salad
- Salmon ramen
- Sweet potato and goats' cheese
- Crispy sea bass and couscous
- Hummus and dips
- Scrambled tofu

05: Yummy snacks and puddings

Week 1 onwards

Celeriac chips

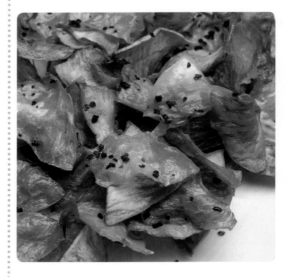

Ingredients
Celeriac
Paprika
Chilli

Preparation method

1 Cut into chip bite sizes, put in the oven with paprika, and chilli if you like it hot, and cook on 190°C for about 30-40 mins.

2 In week 2 you can cover with coconut oil, which is divine.

Week 2-8 and 10-12 (weeks 1 and 9 without oil)

Salt & vinegar kale crisps

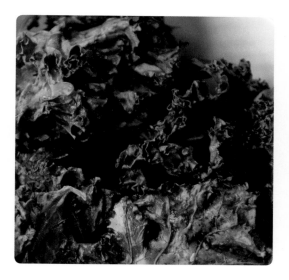

Ingredients
1 large bunch of kale
120g sunflower seeds, finely ground
1 tbsp balsamic vinegar
1 tbsp apple cider vinegar
1 tbsp olive oil
1 tsp salt

Preparation method
1 Combine all the ingredients in a large bowl and mix into the kale.

2 Heat the oven to 150°C. Place a piece of parchment paper on top of a baking sheet, then spread out the kale crisps mixture evenly over the surface.

3 Bake for 2 hours, keeping a close eye as it can burn easily. You can cook the crisps quicker on a higher heat, but they retain more nutrients if you cook them more slowly.

Banana Ice-cream
A really simple recipe, place a banana in a freezer;- it's better out of the skin. Wait for it to freeze and then eat as a delightful ice cream snack.

Week 2 till 9, 10, 11, 12

Nut Loaf
Makes 1 loaf

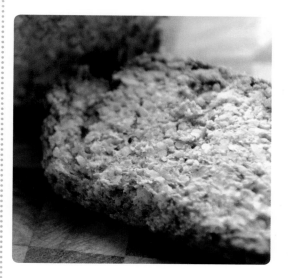

Ingredients
250g of almonds
250g quinoa flakes or uncooked brown rice
300g pumpkin seeds
200g sunflower seeds
2 tbsp chia seeds
3 heaped tbsp psyllium husk powder
2 tbsp dried mixed herbs

Preparation method
1 Place the almonds, quinoa flakes and half the pumpkin seeds in a food processor until smooth.
2 Place this in a bowl with the remaining pumpkin seeds and the sunflower seeds, chia seeds, psyllium husk, dried herbs and salt to taste.
3 Add 3-4 cups of cold water and let the mixture sit for an hour.
4 Heat the oven to 180°C.
5 Once the mixture is really firm grease the base of a loaf tin with coconut or olive oil, pour the mixture in and press it down with a spoon. Bake in the oven for 40 mins to an hour, until the top begins to brown and you can pull a knife out of the middle without any of the mixture sticking to it. Finally, slice, smother on your favourite toppings and enjoy.
6 Storing the bread in the fridge makes it last longer, and you can freeze it, too.

Week 4 till 9, 11, 12

The Body Rescue chocolate goo cake
(flour free, sugar-free)

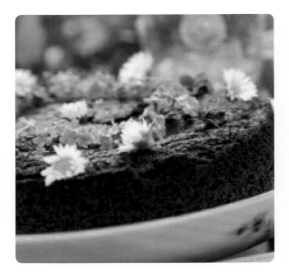

Ingredients
200g coconut oil
4 tbsp chia seeds soaked in a cup of water
for 15 mins.
½ cup raw cocoa
5 medium eggs
1 cup ground almonds
1 cup of natural sweetener (choose coconut or
palm sugar, yacon or Stevia)
Pinch of salt (Celtic or Himalayan)
1 tsp bicarbonate of soda

Preparation method
1 Whisk eggs, then mix with all the ingredients
together in a large bowl.

2 Grease a cake tin and place the mixture in the
tin and bake at 180°C for 45 mins.

3 This is a delicious cake to be eaten warm or
cold.

4 I like to place fruit or edible flowers on top!

Imagine, a cake without sugar or flour – who
would know?

Week 4 till 9, 11, 12

Avocado, banana, carob and honey spread
Serves 1

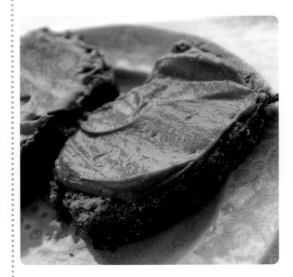

*This rich, creamy spread makes an excellent snack!
Especially good during times of overwork, nervous
tension or strenuous sporting activity.*

Ingredients
½ small ripe banana
¼ large ripe avocado
2 tsp carob powder
1-2 tsp honey
A few drops of real vanilla essence (optional)

Preparation method
1 Peel the banana and the avocado, then mash
them together with the carob powder, honey and
vanilla essence, if using, until you get a creamy
consistency.

2 Spread onto the nut bread in previous recipe.

Weeks 5 till 9 and 11, 12
Orange carrot cream muffins
Makes 12

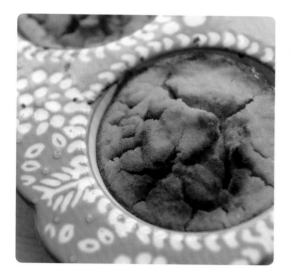

Ingredients
450g rice flour
½ tsp baking soda
¼ tsp baking powder
½ tsp salt
1 tsp cinnamon
1 cup of walnuts, roughly chopped
1 handful of dried fruit
2 tsp ground chia seed
6 tbsp hot water
1 x 400 ml can coconut milk
1 tsp vanilla
14oz fruit pulp, or grate some apple, or carrot

Preparation method
1 Preheat oven to 350°F. Grease muffin pans.

2 Place sifted flour, baking soda, baking powder, salt and cinnamon together in a bowl. Add walnuts and dried fruit.

3 Mix together ground chia and hot water in a separate bowl and then add vanilla and coconut milk.

4 Add the pulp or grated mixture and mix in well, and add half the water.

5 Combine both mixtures. If needed, add the rest of the water.

6 Make muffin shapes, spoon batter into trays, and bake for 30 to 40 mins.

Week 4 till 9, 11, 12
Sweet potato brownies
Makes 5 brownies

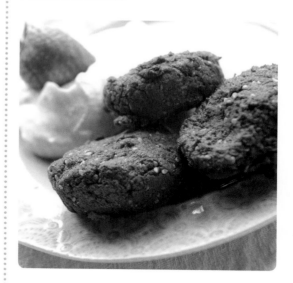

Ingredients
1 sweet potato
1 handful of sesame seeds
120g of ground almonds
60g of buckwheat flour
7 dates
2 tbsp raw cacao
2 tbsp agave nectar
1 pinch of salt

Preparation method
1 Put oven on at 180°C.

2 Peel and cut the sweet potatoes and cook till they are soft (steam or bake).

Add the dates and sweet potato to a blender for a yummy mix.

3 Now add blend all the other ingredients together in with the mix in a bowl.

4 Place in a baking dish and cook for 20 mins.

When you take it out make sure you leave it for at least 10 mins. to cool down or it may fall apart!

Week 4 till 9, 11, 12

Quince and apple crumble
Serves 8

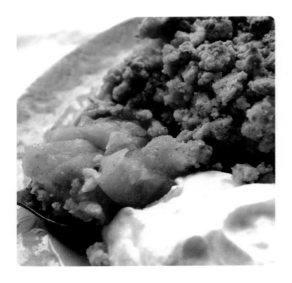

I adore apple crumble and this is an amazing recipe!

Ingredients

4 quince, peeled and cut into eighths (use pears if you cannot get quince)
4 apples
100g raisins
½ tsp ground allspice
½ tsp ground cinnamon
½ tsp sea salt
4 tbsp coconut flour
100ml apple juice

For the crumble topping

150g coconut oil, melted
250g rice flour
100ml agave nectar
½ tsp sea salt
60g chopped nuts

To serve

Natural yogurt

Preparation method

1 Preheat the oven to 190ºC/gas mark 5. Put the quinces in a small saucepan with water and cook for 10 mins.

2 Put the apples, sultanas/golden raisins, allspice, cinnamon, salt, almond flour, apple juice and cooked quince in a mixing bowl. Stir to combine, making sure you turn and coat every piece of fruit. Put the mixture into a 25cm square baking dish. Bake in the preheated oven for 15–20 mins, until the juices are bubbling.

3 Put the coconut oil, flour, agave nectar, salt and pecans in a large bowl. Bring together using your hands, until a sticky dough forms.

4 Remove the baking dish from the oven and scatter the dough randomly over the fruit. Return to the oven and bake for a further 10–15 mins, until the crumble is golden. Allow to cool slightly before serving with a yogurt.

For your convenience there is a 1 week eating plan that you can eat from week 3 (page 114)

And a 7 day menu with shopping list from week 3 till 9, and then 11 & 12 (page 126)

06:

Diet Plan

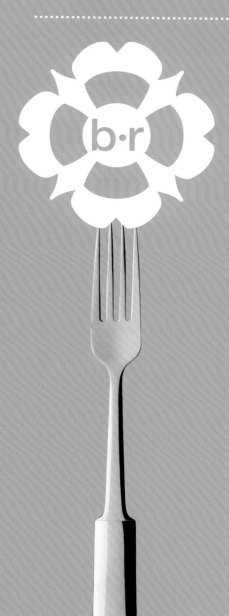

My Diet

I have written this diet so the meals are really quick, easy to make, really tasty and fill you up! If you don't like Nakd Bars, have the equivalent nuts and seeds.

If you don't like seafood have white meat. If you are vegetarian, replace with tofu or soya.

The recipes are written for four people, the menu below is for 1 person.

Shopping list and recipe plan included in this chapter.

Fruit is unlimited!

Monday

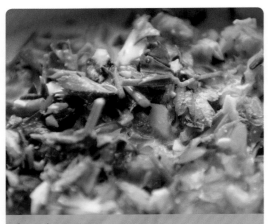

Lunch
Grilled veg. with salsa and potato

Breakfast
Stir fry bananas, 1 handful cashew nuts and raisins in teaspoon of coconut oil and add to unlimited plain low fat yogurt, top with tbsp of milled flaxseed and tbsp agave nectar.

Lunch
Grilled veg. with salsa and potato
(see recipe)

Supper
Spaghetti with tomato and courgette sauce
(see recipe)

Snack
Fruit and one handful of seeds, nuts and dried fruit. 1 Nakd Bar

JUICE OF THE DAY
Carrots, 3 strawberries, 1 passion fruit, ½ red cabbage.

Tuesday

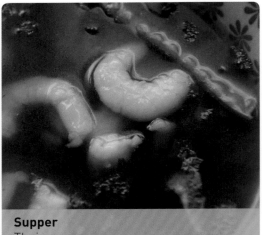

Supper
Thai prawn soup

Breakfast
Plain low fat yogurt, fruit, 1 handful milled flaxseed

Lunch
Fish pie
(see recipe)

Supper
Thai prawn soup
(see recipe)

Snack
1 Nakd Bar or nuts and seeds plus fruit.

JUICE OF THE DAY
Carrot, apple and ginger

Wednesday

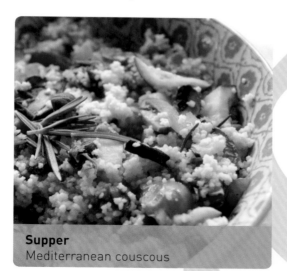

Supper
Mediterranean couscous

Breakfast
Banana omelette
(see recipe)

Lunch
½ Jacket potato and smoked salmon and salad

Supper
Mediterranean couscous

Snack
1 Nakd Bar plus fruit and handful of dried fruit

JUICE OF THE DAY
Grape juice

Thursday

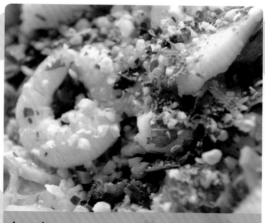

Lunch
Mango and prawn salad

Breakfast
Yogurt, fruit and 1 handful of milled flaxseed

Lunch
Mango and prawn salad
(see recipe)

Supper
Butternut squash and chilli risotto
(see recipe)

Snack
1 Nakd Bar and fruit

JUICE OF THE DAY
1 orange, 1 apple, 1 carrot, 1 grapefruit and 1 pear

Friday

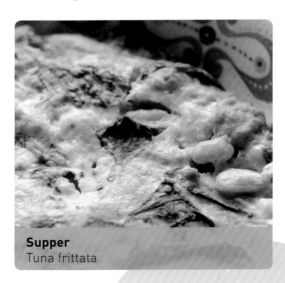

Supper
Tuna frittata

Breakfast
60g of Porridge with yoghurt and fruit

Lunch
Jacket potato and ½ can of baked beans
(sugar free).
Handful of grated cheese and 1 tbs. olive oil.

Supper
Tuna frittata
(see recipe)

Snack
1 Nakd Bar and fruit

JUICE OF THE DAY
Carrot, apple and ginger

Saturday

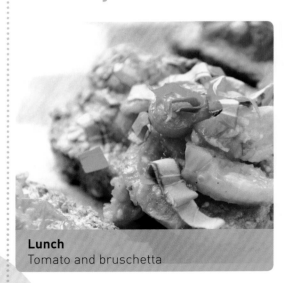

Lunch
Tomato and bruschetta

Breakfast
60g of Porridge with yoghurt and fruit

Lunch
Tomato and bruschetta
(see recipe)

Supper
Creamy vegetable dahl
(see recipe)

Snack
1 Nakd Bar and fruit

JUICE OF THE DAY
Grape juice

Sunday

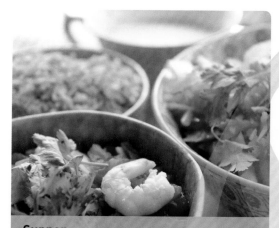

Supper
Vegetable balti and prawn curry

Breakfast
Banana omelette
(see recipe)

Lunch
Steamed salmon with coconut sauce
(see recipe)

Supper
Vegetable balti and prawn curry
(see recipe)

Snack
Fruit

JUICE OF THE DAY
1 orange, 1 apple, 1 carrot, 1 grapefruit
and 1 pear

7 day Body Rescue
Diet Plan recipes

b·r

Diet plan recipes | Monday
Grilled veg. with salsa and potato

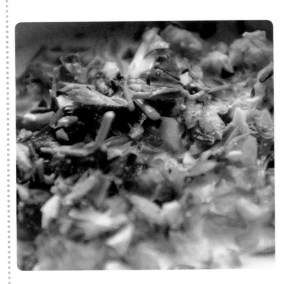

Ingredients
1 red pepper
1 yellow pepper
2 red onions
3 courgettes
14 cherry tomatoes
Olive oil
2 garlic cloves
½ tsp dried red chilli flakes
1tbsp rosemary leaves, finely chopped
1tbsp thyme leaves

For the herb salsa
3 tbsp flat leaf parsley
2 tbsp snipped chives
1 garlic clove
1 lemon
150ml. water
1 tbsp fromage frais
salt and pepper

TO GARNISH
Rosemary sprigs

Preparation method
1 First make the salsa by placing all the ingredients in a food processor until smooth and then season.

2 Cut the peppers into bite-sized chunks and the

red onion into thin wedges, whilst cutting the courgettes into thick slices. Put the vegetables and cherry tomatoes in a large bowl and add some oil. Add the garlic and chilli flakes , rosemary and thyme. Season and toss to mix. Preheat the grill.

3 Place the vegetables under the grill for 10 mins until lightly charred.

4 To serve, place vegetables on 4 plates and drizzle over salsa. Add some rosemary and a jacket potato if you prefer.

Spaghetti with tomato and courgette sauce

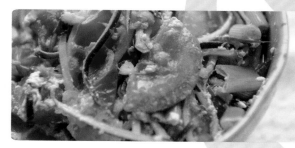

Ingredients
200g/7oz cherry tomatoes
1 courgette trimmed
350g/12oz dried spaghetti
1 tbsp coconut oil
1 garlic clove, peeled and crushed
1 bunch basil
2 tbsp fromage frais
6 spring onions, finely sliced
Salt and black pepper

TO GARNISH
Basil

Preparation method
1 Cut half the tomatoes and place half to reserve. Grate the courgettes.

2 Cook the spaghetti according to instructions.

4 Chop the basil and place in a bowl with the fromage frais, spring onions and chopped tomatoes. Stir and add to the frying pan.

5 Serve the spaghetti and sauce together and eat immediately.

Diet Plan recipes | Tuesday
Fish pie

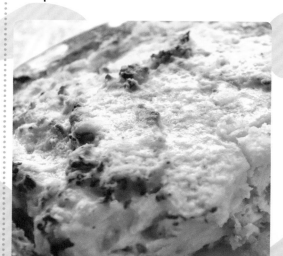

Ingredients
500g potatoes, diced
1 medium swede cut into chunks
200g soft cheese with herbs
150ml vegetable stock
650g skinless, boneless cod, cut into large chunks
100g cooked peeled prawns
1 tsp chopped fresh parsley
Cheese

Preparation method
1 Boil the potatoes and swede until tender for 20 mins.

2 Preheat the oven to 190°C/ gas 5/fan 170°C. Put the soft cheese and stock into a large saucepan and heat gently until smooth.

3 Stir the fish into the sauce with the prawns and parsley.

4 Put the mixture into a baking dish. Drain the potatoes and swede, mash them well and season with black pepper. Spoon the mash over the fish to cover it completely. Bake for 25-30 mins, then grate some cheese and add to the top and grill for 5 mins.

Serve with vegetables of your choice.

Thai prawn soup

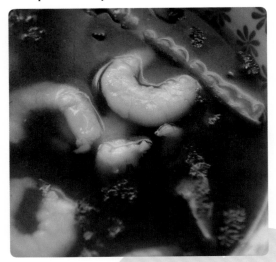

Mediterranean couscous

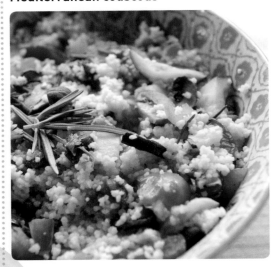

Ingredients

8 spring onions, finely shredded
2 fresh lemongrass stalks, very finely shredded
1 garlic clove, peeled and crushed
1 inch finely grated fresh root ginger
½ red chilli, deseeded and finely sliced
900ml/1½ pts of stock
60g/2oz shiitake mushrooms
60g/2oz mangetout
200g/7oz raw tiger prawns, peeled and deveined
1tbsp dark soya sauce (sugar free)
Vegetable stock or Miso soup
Handful of chopped coriander leaves

Preparation method

1 Place the spring onions, lemongrass, garlic, ginger, chilli and stock in a large saucepan, cover and bring to the boil.

2 Add the mushrooms and mangetout to the pan. Cook for 3mins then add the prawns and soya sauce. Cook for a further 2-3 mins. until the prawns turn pink. Take off the heat.

3 Stir in the coriander and serve straight away.

Ingredients

Coconut oil
1 large red pepper
1 yellow pepper
6 baby courgettes
2 red onions
4 large mushrooms
8-10 medium tomatoes
3 tbsp chopped rosemary leaves
250g/9oz couscous
450ml/1pint boiling hot veg. stock or water
2 garlic cloves, peeled and finely grated
3 tbsp chopped flat leaf parsley
100g/3½oz capers or caper berries
salt and pepper

Preparation method

1 Preheat oven 200°C/ gas 6/fan 180°C. Cut the peppers into bite sized chunks and add into a large roasting tin with oil along with the courgettes, onions, mushrooms and tomatoes. Sprinkle with the rosemary and roast in the oven for 15 mins.

2 Put the couscous in a large bowl add water until cooked.

3 Mix the garlic and lemon together in a bowl add the couscous the roasted veg. Add the garlic and lemon, chopped herbs and capers. Season and toss.

Banana omelette

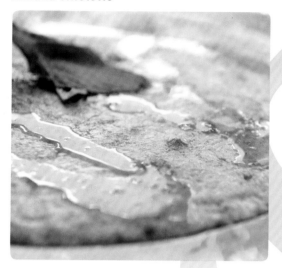

A delicious alternative to pancakes!

Ingredients
2 large bananas
4 eggs
1 large pinch of cinnamon

Preparation method
1 Mash the bananas well in a bowl.

2 Add the cinnamon and mix well.

3 Whisk the eggs and add.

4 Cook on a pan, serve, enjoy!

Mango and prawn salad

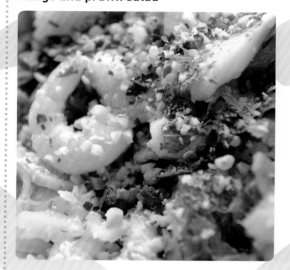

Ingredients
Cooked, peeled prawns - preferably large ones
1 large ripe mango, diced
4 tbsp vegetable oil
4 shallots, finely sliced
chopped mint leaves
chopped coriander leaves
100g toasted chopped cashews (unsalted)

Dressing
125ml rice vinegar
Crushed clove of garlic
1 small dried red chilli, crushed
Juice of a large lime - Fish sauce to taste

Preparation method
1 Bring the vinegar to the boil. Remove from the heat, add garlic and chilli and leave to cool.

2 Add lime juice, and a few drops of fish sauce to taste.

3 Fry shallots in oil until brown and crispy, being careful not to let them burn. Drain on kitchen paper and reserve the oil. Leave to cool. The recipe so far can be made in advance.

4 Then, just before you're ready to serve, combine the prawns, mango and herbs and toss with a drizzle of the oil and a good lashing of the dressing.

5 Put into small serving dishes and scatter the cashews and shallots over the top.

Butternut squash and chilli risotto

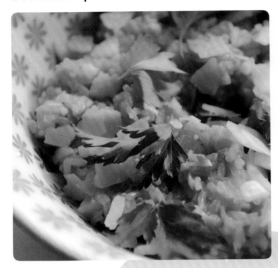

Tuna frittata

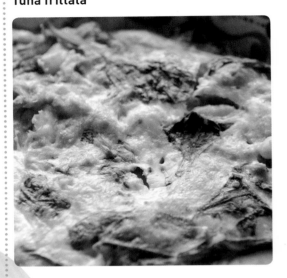

Ingredients
coconut oil
900ml/1½pints vegetable stock
1 finely chopped red onion
2 garlic cloves, finely chopped
1 red chilli, finely chopped
255g/9oz of arborio or risotto rice
140g/5oz chopped butternut squash
3 tbsp. flat leaf parsley 30g/1oz parmesan

Preparation method
1 Bring the stock to the boil in a saucepan and add rice.

2 Meanwhile add coconut oil to a wok or frying pan.

3 Fry red onion, garlic and 1 chilli, and cook gently for 2-3 mins, stirring occasionally.

4 Add butternut squash and vegetables to the stock and keep stirring until cooked.

Ingredients
2 cans tuna in vegetable oil.
400g cannellini beans, rinsed, well-drained
175g cheese, grated
1 handful spinach leaves
1 tsp dried oregano
8 eggs, lightly beaten
2½ tbsp. coconut oil
salt and pepper to season

Preparation method
1 Place tuna, beans, cheese, spinach leaves and oregano in a large bowl, add the eggs and mix well, season to taste.

2 Add the egg mixture in a large frying pan with heated oil and cook for 2-3 mins. Using a spatula slightly lift around the edges to allow some of the uncooked mixture to run under the sides. Cook for another 2-3 mins, or until it is set around the edges, but still soft in the middle.

3 Turn the frittata over and cook for 3 mins. Remove from the heat and allow the frittata to stand for 5 mins in the pan.

4 Serve with a crunchy salad.

Tomato and bruschetta

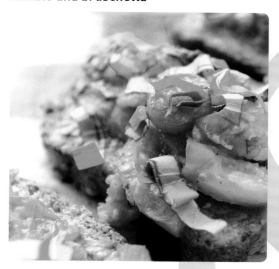

Creamy vegetable dahl

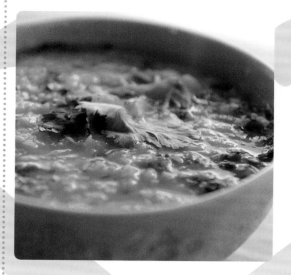

Ingredients

7 plum tomatoes, 2 cloves garlic, minced, 1 tbsp extra virgin olive oil, 1 tsp balsamic vinegar, 1tsp cider vinegar

6-8 fresh basil leaves, chopped

salt and freshly ground black pepper to taste

1/4 cup olive oil

Nut loaf bread (see nut loaf recipe)

Preparation method sauce

1 Boil the tomatoes for one minute drain and remove the skins.

Cut them in quarters and remove the seeds and juice from their centres.

2 Preheat the oven to 450°F 230°C/ gas 8 /fan 210°C

3 While the oven is heating, chop up the tomatoes finely. Put tomatoes, garlic, 1 tbsp extra virgin olive oil, vinegar in a bowl and mix. Add the chopped basil. Add salt and pepper to taste.

4 Slice the nut loaf bread thickly, Coat one side of each slice with olive oil using a pastry brush and rub some garlic onto it too.

5 Place a tray of bread slices in the oven on the top rack. Toast for 5-6 mins, until the bread just begins to turn golden brown.

6 Place the bread on a serving platter, olive oil side up, place some topping on each slice of bread and serve. If you top each slice with the tomatoes, do it right before serving or the bread may get soggy.

Ingredients

350g split red lentils, 1tsp ground turmeric

2 large fresh green chillies chopped,

1tbsp coconut oil, 1tsp brown mustard seeds,

1tsp cumin seeds, 2tsp garam masala

1tsp ground coriander

125mls (½ cup) water

1 large ripe tomato, chopped

salt & ground black pepper, to taste

1/4 cup chopped fresh coriander

Preparation method

1 Combine the lentils, split peas, turmeric and chillies to a large saucepan of boiling water and boil, uncovered, for 30 mins, until tender. Drain and place in a bowl. Mash roughly with a fork and set aside.

2 Heat the coconut oil in the saucepan over medium heat and cook the mustard seeds and cumin seeds for 30 seconds or until the mustard seeds begin to pop. Add the garam masala and coriander and cook for 30 seconds.

3 Add in the lentils and peas, water, and tomato and bring to the boil, reduce heat to low and simmer, partially covered, stirring often, for 4 mins.

4 Stir in the coriander and serve immediately.

Diet Plan recipes | Sunday

Steamed coconut salmon

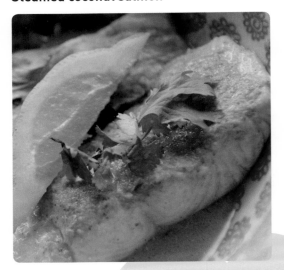

Vegetable balti and prawn curry

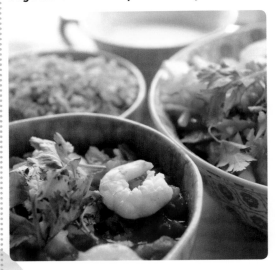

Ingredients
4 salmon fillets, skinned
salt and freshly ground black pepper

For the marinade:
2tbsp coconut milk
2 green chillies, deseeded and finely diced
2tbsp chopped coriander leaves
2 garlic cloves, peeled and crushed
2tsp finely grated fresh root ginger
Juice of 1 lemon 100ml (3½ fl oz) hot water

TO GARNISH
lemon wedges coriander leaves

Preparation method
1 Place all the marinade ingredients in a food processor and blend until fairly smooth. Transfer to a bowl.

2 Add all the marinade to the salmon and steam or grill for about 15-20 mins until it flakes

3 Serve garnished with lemon wedges and coriander leaves.

Vegetable balti

Ingredients
3 large carrots, peeled
1 swede, peeled
1 onion, peeled and finely chopped
300g (10oz) green beans, trimmed and halved
1 red pepper, cored, deseeded and roughly chopped
300ml (½pt) vegetable stock
2 garlic cloves, peeled and grated
1tsp finely grated fresh root ginger
1tbsp medium curry powder
400g (14oz) can chopped tomatoes
Salt and freshly ground black pepper
4tbsp chopped coriander leaves

To serve
Coriander sprigs to garnish, lemon or lime wedges, very low fat natural yogurt.

Preparation method
1 Cut the carrots and swede into bite-sized chunks and place in a large saucepan with the onion, green beans and red pepper. Add the stock, garlic, ginger and curry powder. Bring to the boil and cook over a medium heat for 8-10 mins, stirring occasionally.

2 Stir in the chopped tomatoes and season, bringing back to the boil. Simmer, uncovered, for 5-6 mins.

3 Let the balti stand for 5 mins, then stir in the chopped coriander.

Serve immediately, garnished with coriander sprigs. Accompany with natural yogurt,

lemon or lime wedges, and steamed or boiled rice.

Prawn Curry

Ingredients
2tbsp curry paste (sugar free)
1 onion, finely sliced
200g large raw prawns
400g can chopped tomatoes garlic
large bunch coriander, leaves and stalks chopped

Preparation method
1 Gently heat some oil into a wok or frying pan, then add the onion for 4 mins. until the onion softens, then stir in the paste and cook for a few mins. longer. Stir in the prawns and tomatoes, then bring to a simmer.

2 Simmer prawns until they have changed colour and are cooked through. Season and then add the coriander just before serving with the vegetable balti.

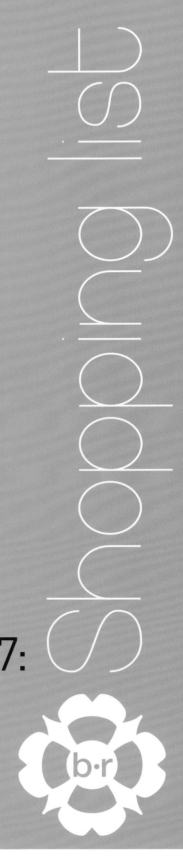

07: Shopping list

Vegetables, herbs and spices

1 can of baked beans (sugar free)

400g can chopped tomatoes with garlic

5 large carrots, peeled

3 swedes, peeled

300g (10oz) green beans

400g (14oz) can chopped tomatoes

200g (7oz) frozen peas

1 large ripe tomato

2 onions

2 carrots

½ red cabbage

4 courgettes

12 cherry tomatoes in olive oil

200g/ 7oz cherry tomatoes

16 garlic cloves

1 chopped butternut squash

12 spring onions

2 large red pepper

1 yellow pepper

6 baby courgettes

4 red onions, peeled and quartered

4 large mushrooms, thickly sliced

8-10 medium tomatoes on the vine

6 or 7 ripe plum tomatoes (about 1½ lbs)

4 red chillies

vegetable stock

60g/ 2oz shiitake mushrooms

60g/ 2oz mangetout

baby spinach leaves

2 fresh lemongrass stalks

3 tbsp chopped rosemary leaves

1tsp dried oregano

½tsp crushed dried red chilli flakes

1tbsp rosemary leaves, finely chopped

1tsbp thyme leaves

10tbsp. flat leaf parsley

2tbsp chives

rosemary sprigs

2 bunch basil

1tsp chopped fresh parsley

12tbsp coriander leaves

1 large pinch of cinnamon

4 shallots

finely sliced mint leaves

1tsp ground turmeric

2 large fresh green chillies

1tsp brown mustard seeds

1tsp cumin seeds

2tsp garam masala

1tsp ground coriander

2 ginger

Dairy

1 tub of fromage frais

200g tub of soft cheese with garlic and herbs

12 eggs

1 packet cheddar

60g/ 2oz parmesan.

2 tubs of natural yogurt

Sauces

Virgin olive oil

coconut oil

125ml rice vinegar

fish sauce

1tbsp medium curry powder

1tbsp dark soya sauce

balsamic vinegar

cider vinegar

agave nectar

150ml vegetable stock

Carbs

spaghetti

500g potatoes

250g/ 9oz couscous

255g/ 9oz. of arborio or risotto rice

porridge oats

jacket potato

quinoa flakes

Fish

650g skinless, boneless cod

100g cooked peeled prawns

200g/ 7oz raw tiger prawns, peeled

2 (195g) cans tuna in vegetable oil

4 salmon fillets, each about 200g (7oz), skinned

200g large raw or cooked prawns

Fruit

100g/3½oz capers or caper berries

4 big bananas

1 lime

2 lemon

2 orange

4 apple

1 can of coconut milk

2 grapefruit

2 pear

1 bunch of grapes

3 strawberries

1 passion fruit

1 large ripe mango

Nuts, seeds, beans and pulses

200g toasted chopped cashews (unsalted)

400g cannellini beans, rinsed, well-drained

350g split red lentils

1 bag of milled flaxseeds

250g of almonds

300g pumpkin seeds

200g sunflower seeds

2 tbsp chia seeds

3 heaped tbsp psyllium husk powder

2 tbsp dried mixed herbs

Other

Nakd Bars

''You gotta have a body.''
Jayne Mansfield

Chapter 8
The Body Rescue Exercise Plan

01: Why exercise?

02: The best way to burn fat

03: The quickest workout

04: Choosing exercises

05: Warm-up exercises

06: Abdominal workout 1

07: Explanation of moves

08: Cardiovascular training

09: Interval training 1

10: Explanation of moves

11: Resistance workout 1

12: Explanation of moves

13: Abdominal workout 2

14: Explanation of moves

15: Interval training 2

16: Explanation of moves

17: Resistance workout 2

18: Explanation of moves

19: Stretch

20: Exercise programme

The Body Rescue Exercise Plan Introduction

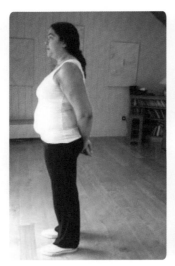
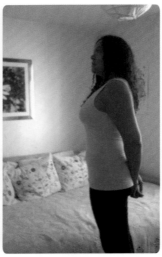
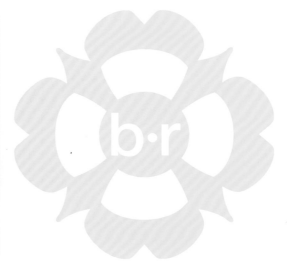

This is my amazing client, Daniella. She lost 2.5 stone in 10 weeks whilst doing my Body Rescue Plan – and is such an inspiration.

When you consider losing weight, it's not just about the aesthetics, it's about how else it is affecting you and ageing you. Daniella had terrible back problems before she started training with me, you can see that the pull from her enlarged tummy would create strain on her back. Her face also has a grey tone to it, despite her having naturally dark skin, and is swollen; even her eyes look sullen and grey. In the 'after' photo Daniella not only looks about 15 years younger, but her back pain went and she got her health, vigour and confidence back, which made her feel that much younger too. Like most of us, Daniella is busy and needed a plan that fitted in with her lifestyle, she is a working mum of two young children, but still managed to fit my easy plan into her life and have incredible results.

This was only in 10 weeks, no gimmicks, no slimming drinks, no weighing and measuring, no points, no counting calories or looking at fat, just my simple plan changed her life!

I actually bumped into Daniella recently and she came up to me in the street saying that I have changed her life forever and the weight had stayed off two years on, this is music to my ears and I never grow tired of knowing I can be the catalyst to improving, empowering and energising someone's life.

01: Why exercise?

Exercise...

- **Lowers your blood pressure**
- **Makes you live longer**
- **Lowers your pulse**
- **Strengthens and tones you**
- **Makes your skin look younger**
- **Improves your heart and lung function**
- **Improves your circulation**
- **Helps you lose weight**
- **Increases your libido**
- **Helps you combat stress**
- **Rids depression**
- **Lifts your mood**
- **Makes you look, feel and be fit**
- **Increases your confidence**
- **Improves your sleep**
- **To name but a few...**

Mindset with exercise.
I have mentioned quite a bit about tapping into your positive mindset and continually perfecting it to maintain and strengthen your mind like a muscle would grow. I have also mentioned limiting beliefs and how they can pull you back from your goals. The other thing you may want to consider is how to set the day up to create and manipulate the environment around you so you feel like exercising and eating well.

Personally, music really creates a mood for me
– if I go for a jog and I am feeling tired, then blasting my ears with some dance music always works, every time. If I already have good energy, I love the sound of nature and focussing and absorbing the beautiful energies around me.

Equally, if am stressed and want to meditate I set the mood so that my mind feels calm
– this works well for my clients, too! Whenever ever I teach an evening yoga and meditation class at my Body Rescue fitness and well being centre, I set the mood, relaxation music, lights dimmed, and candles lit around the room, so the moment my clients walk in, they switch off from whatever day they have had and feel serene. I always get told that yoga nights are the nights my clients get their best night's sleep.

Even smells can change your mood, if you are trying to relax;
then burning incense or scented candles can make you go from stressed to calm the moment you light them.

It's about touching all your senses for stimulus, sight, sound, smell, taste, and touch.

Clothes can also make you feel in a uniform for working out or relaxing.
If we work, we put on our work clothes, suits can make people feel empowered, trendy clothes can make people feel sexy, colourful clothes can make you feel bright and dressing for a black tie event can make you feel glamorous.

Equally, workout clothes can make you feel like working out, and snuggly warm clothes can make you feel relaxed for a meditation. Just imagine how you would feel wearing a suit for a meditation – it would trigger work thoughts and you would find it hard to unwind – or just imagine going to a business meeting in your snuggly clothes, you would feel like falling asleep.

We all have uniforms that make us feel like getting on with that job, they set the mindset. So get yourself some practical and gorgeous workout gear that makes you feel like a sexy athlete the moment it goes on. Once those clothes are on, I doubt you would then go and eat a chocolate cake, it would inspire you to get up and go.

Being accountable to someone can also inspire you stick to a plan, so why not find a workout friend that you can both help on your journey?
I would advise not to use your partner for this as it could lead to rows and over-expectations!

What makes you want to exercise?

_____

_____

_____

If you were knackered, what would make you spring up?

_____

_____

_____

How you can create an environment that would make you want to exercise?

_____

_____

_____

Again, create your own fitness advert that has subliminal messages!

02: The best way to burn fat

Definitions...

Cardiovascular training
Training your heart and lungs at a consistent level for Interval training.

Calories
A calorie is a unit of energy, we need calories as energy in food to live. Around 2500 for men and 2000 for women a day.

Metabolism
Metabolism converts the fuel in the food we eat into the energy needed to power everything we do, from moving to thinking to growing.
Carbs- Carb is short for carbohydrate, a component of food that is used mainly for energy in the body. Good carbs are brown rice, whole meal pasta, couscous, fruit, vegetables, potatoes, not good carbs are biscuits, white bread etc.

....

Calories burned in exercise

I do not mention calories much in this book, as it is not always entirely relevant.
The old rule was eat around 1500 calories a day for a woman to lose weight and 2000 for a man to lose weight.

Or consume 1800 calories for a woman for maintenance or 2500 calories for a man.

Recent research has proven that calories are not all equal,
if you lived of a diet of 1500 calories of crisps and chocolate, chances are you would actually put on weight because of the effects on your hormones and insulin levels, not to mention the catastrophic effect on your poor digestion and all your organ function, joints, muscles, oh. and your skin, hair and even eyeballs would probably look awful too.

However, every time you exercise, you do burn calories, which in turn can lead to your fat melting away.
The amount of calories you burn depends on the specific exercise you are doing, how intense it is and how long you do it for.

....

Calories burned after the workout helps fat burning.

The more intense the exercise you perform, the more your overall metabolism is boosted and the more calories your body will burn after the workout.

If you only do slow cardio training for your fat loss, you will burn calories during the workout, but your metabolism will go back to its normal rate soon after.
The way you can actually raise your metabolism for up to 24 hours after, is by doing interval training as you create a much greater demand on your body.

Your hormonal response to exercise affects fat loss.
When you exercise, your body secretes hormones in response to the training. The key one that you want to work on for fat loss is growth hormone (GH)

One of the main functions of GH is to send a signal to your body to burn fat for fuel and one of the ways we maximise the release of natural GH in the body from training is lactic acid.

When the body detects large amounts of lactic acid in the blood stream GH is released in response. **So the more intense the exercise and burn, the greater the GH release.**

It is for this reason I have included Interval training (as below) as part of your fitness plan; however, as this is very intensive, we just do this just 1-2 times a week.

When doing Interval style training, you will get the better effect by performing this training on an empty stomach.
This is because GH secretion is reduced by both elevated blood sugar levels and elevated insulin levels in the body.

When you eat something your blood sugar will rise and insulin will be secreted as a result.
Insulin is a storage hormone and works directly against GH. (However, if you feel faint training on an empty stomach or need some food for energy, please don't worry too much about this as you will work harder with food! This does not apply to cardiovascular training, you will need something to eat before that, as lactic acid is not released in cardio and you are training for a longer period of time.)

After training Interval style you can consume carbs and it won't affect the post-workout fat-burning process. Your body will continue to use stored fat to fuel the workout even when you take in carbs.

Cardiovascular training, yoga, Pilates and meditation are also all really beneficial and part of my body rescue fitness plan.
All these exercises will give you an all-round training, burning fat, lengthening your limbs, calming your mind, and not putting too much stress on the body, but sculpting it to perfection.

The hormone cortisol can relate to how you hold your belly fat.
Your body will produce cortisol (and encourage belly fat storage) under conditions of nearly any type of stress – both emotional and physical – **so rather than creating too much cardio, it is of far greater effect to combat cortisol through resistance training. Cortisol has been linked to overtraining and has a catabolic (muscle wasting) effect.**

Short, intense training sessions will help to counteract the effects of cortisol;
both the muscle wasting effect, and the cortisol related belly fat storage, and yoga/meditation style exercises will help, too.

And traditional style Pilates exercises are better for sculpting your abs than endless sit ups.

03: The quickest workout

The most effective and quickest workout you can do is Interval training.

The full Interval training programme is four minutes long, a very intense four minutes!

Don't underestimate this workout!

Interval training follow this structure:
- Push hard for 20 seconds
- **Rest for 10 seconds.**
- Repeat this eight times.

To make this really effective you have to go for it in those 20 seconds – so do as many reps as you can in the 20 seconds – there is a 10 second rest between each exercise.
If you are a beginner, allow your body time to adjust to this type of exercise, making sure you perform the exercise correctly in the first instance and then once your performance is correct and you feel able, push yourself more.

I would suggest getting some sort of Interval training timer, like a watch where you can see exactly where you are in the workout, or you can buy apps;
you don't want to have to think too much, all of your concentration will be on the exercise.

Interval training exercises

1) 20 seconds running on spot
   10 second rest

2) 20 seconds press up
   10 second rest

3) 20 second lunge walk
   10 second rest

4) 20 second tricep dip
   10 second rest

5) 20 second prisoner
   10 second rest

6) 20 second shuttle run
   10 second rest

7) 20 second lunge kick
   10 second rest

8) 20 second burpee
   10 second rest

04: Choosing exercises

I have suggested two different Interval training routines, one for weeks 3-7 and a more advanced one for weeks 8-12. I know you can do it, you will be very fit by then.

This is not a daily workout; if you can do this every day you are doing it wrong.
I recommend you use this once a week, from week 3.

05: Warm-up exercises

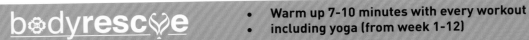

bodyrescue

- Warm up 7-10 minutes with every workout
- including yoga (from week 1-12)

Roll Shoulders

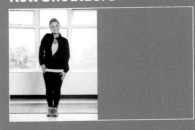

Flex elbows

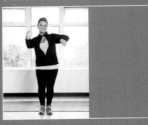

Circle wrists

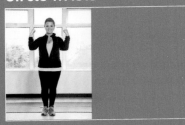

Circle hips

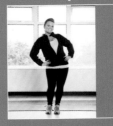

Roll neck

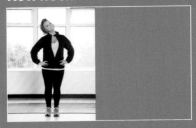

Arch and round your back

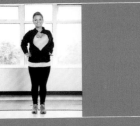

March on the spot

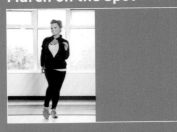

Knees up

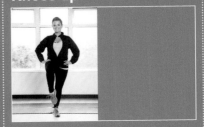

Fast walk or jog: 5 mins

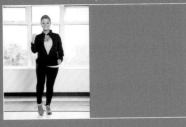

'Your body is the church where
Nature asks to be reverenced.''
Marquis de Sade

- **Roll each joint 5 times in each direction.**

Bend knees

Circle ankles

Run on the spot: 2-3 mins

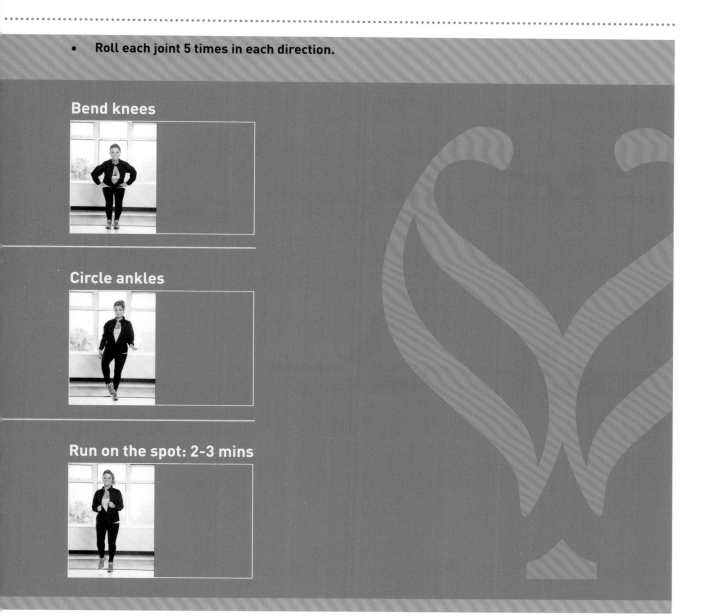

06: Abdominal workout 1

Every day (from week 1-7)

![bodyrescue]

Superman

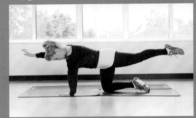

Lean back and twist

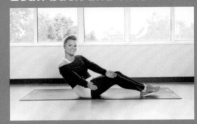

Pullins

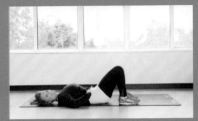

Bridge

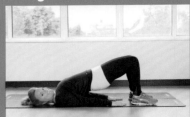

Reverse curl

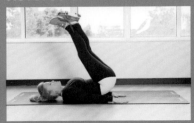

07: Explanation of moves

Superman

Go on all fours, pull your stomach in, stretch your spine, raise your right arm and your left leg at hip height. Reach as far you as can, then lower back down again, together. Breathe out when you raise and breathe in when you lower, trying to keep the hips still.

Lean back and twist

Sit with your knees bent and your feet on the floor. Take your arms out in front of you and lean back about 10 inches, then twist your arms and your whole torso to the right on the exhale. Then breathe in to the front and sit up straight again. Repeat to the other side.

Pullins

Lie on your back (or you can do this standing), breathe out and pull the abs in, as if you are doing up a really tight pair of trousers. Breathe in to release and repeat, focussing on pulling your stomach in like a corset that wraps around you.

Bridge

Lie on your back, knees bent, feet on the floor. Lift your hips off the floor, slowly, and then lower back down, vertebra by vertebra. As you raise, lift your hips and pull your abs in, trying to create the motion through your stomach muscles.

Reverse curls

Lie on your back. Lift your legs in the air. Raise your bottom and lower back off the floor, and then back down again. Don't use your hands on the floor to help you, and don't push into your head. Lower down as gently as you can.

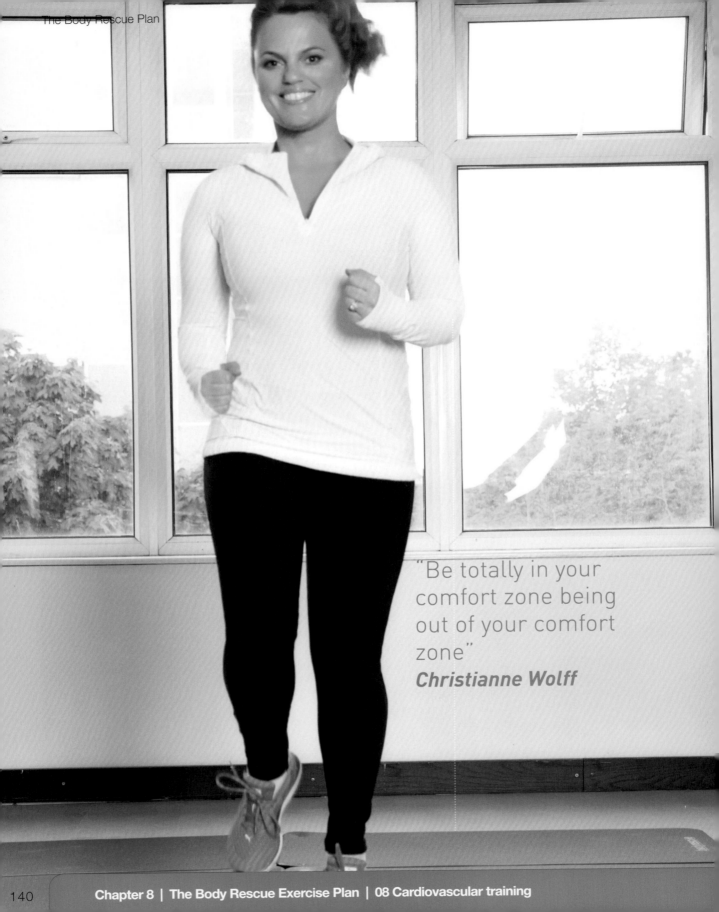

"Be totally in your comfort zone being out of your comfort zone"
Christianne Wolff

08: Cardiovascular training

3 times a week (from week 2)

bodyrescue

The key to sticking to any programme that is different to your routine already, is to get organised!

- Write in your diary where you will fit the exercise in and plan like it is a meeting. Find your diary in chapter 10

- Plan out your week's food in advance, and what meals you will have, so that you are really excited to eat them.

When you perform cardiovascular moves, keep your breathing and pulse at a steady rate, always warming up for 10 minutes and cooling down with a stretch.

Alter the cardio, don't do the same thing each time as your body will get used to it.

To download a new diary go to www.thebodyrescueplan.com

09: Interval training 1

Once a week (from week 3-7)

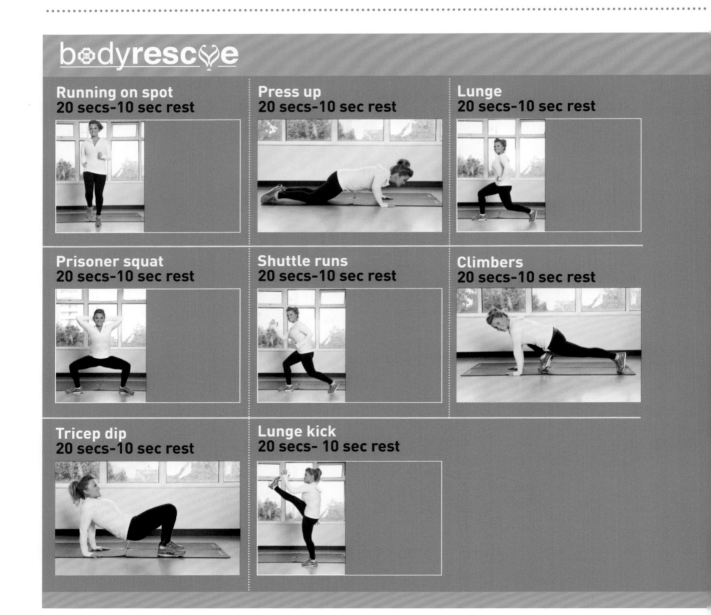

bodyrescue

Running on spot 20 secs-10 sec rest	**Press up** 20 secs-10 sec rest	**Lunge** 20 secs-10 sec rest
Prisoner squat 20 secs-10 sec rest	**Shuttle runs** 20 secs-10 sec rest	**Climbers** 20 secs-10 sec rest
Tricep dip 20 secs-10 sec rest	**Lunge kick** 20 secs- 10 sec rest	

10: Explanation of moves

Running on the spot

Jog or walk on the spot

Press up

Go on your knees and take your hands out on the floor, slightly wider than your hips. Push your hips forward, elbows out to the side and lower your chest to the floor. Don't allow your back to arch, pull your stomach in. Lower as far as you are able, pushing your chest closer to the floor and then back up again. Repeat.

Lunge

Stand, take your right leg forward in a long stride. Place it on the floor and bend both of your knees. Make sure your front leg is at a right angle and your knee is not over your toe. Your back knee should be close to the floor, and your heel up. Now take your left leg forwards and repeat the walk.

Prisoner squat

Take your feet wide apart, with your feet turned out. Bend your knees and push through your heels. Take your hands behind your head and lower your legs and raise, keeping your back up straight.

Shuttle runs

Short sprints in a straight line.

Climbers

Kneel and take your hands on the floor. Take your right knee into your chest, and keep your left leg straight. Alternate, making a fast motion one in one back.

Tricep dip

Sit on the floor or on a chair. Elbows behind you. Lift your hips up in the air and lower your elbows, you should feel this one in the back of the arms straight away. Bend and straighten.

Lunge kick

Same position as the lunge walk description, the back leg goes up in the air into a kick and then back behind again, repeat. Do right and left.

11: Resistance workout 1

Once a week (from week 3-7)

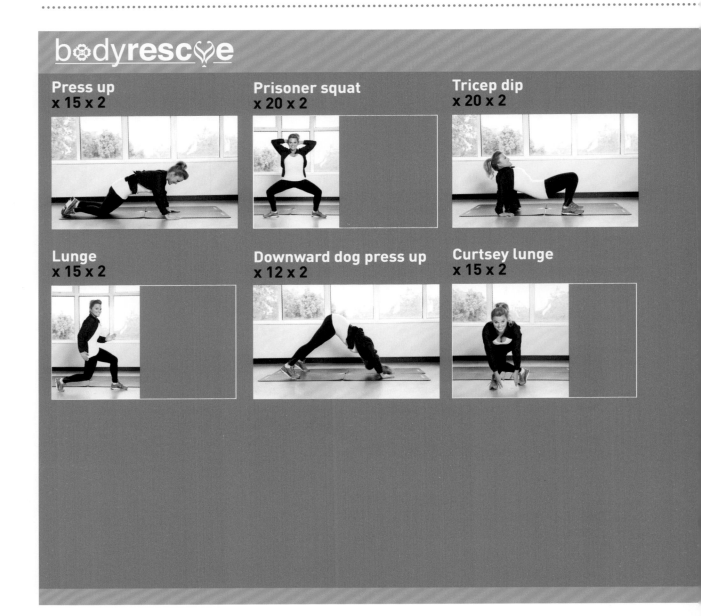

bodyrescue

Press up
x 15 x 2

Prisoner squat
x 20 x 2

Tricep dip
x 20 x 2

Lunge
x 15 x 2

Downward dog press up
x 12 x 2

Curtsey lunge
x 15 x 2

12: Explanation of moves

Press up

Go on your knees and take your hands out on the floor, slightly wider than your hips. Push your hips forward, elbows out to the side and lower your chest to the floor. Don't allow your back to arch, pull your stomach in. Lower as far as you are able, pushing your chest closer to the floor and then back up again. Repeat.

Prisoner squat

Take your feet wide apart, with your feet turned out. Bend your knees and push through your heels. Take your hands behind your head and lower your legs and raise, keeping your back up straight.

Tricep dip

Sit on the floor or on a chair. Elbows behind you. Lift your hips up in the air and lower your elbows, you should feel this one in the back of the arms straight away. Bend and straighten.

Lunge

Stand, take your right leg forward in a long stride. Place it on the floor, and bend both of your knees. Make sure your front leg is at a right angle and your knee is not over your toe. Your back knee should be close to the floor, and your heel up. Take your back knee off the floor and straighten leg, repeat going down again. Do right and left.

Downward dog press up

Stand, and take your hands to the floor. Walk your feet back so that you create a triangle shape, with your bottom in the air and your hands and feet on the floor. Take your elbows out the side and press down towards the floor, feeling the movement in your shoulders. Straighten your arms back up again, make sure your head isn't looking up.

Curtsey lunge

Stand and take your right foot behind the left leg and bend your knees down towards the floor. Take your hands towards your left foot, leaning down to the floor. Come up and take your right knee in the air and your arms in the air, then repeat back to the floor again.
Repeat right and left.

13: Abdominal workout 2

Every day (from week 8-12)

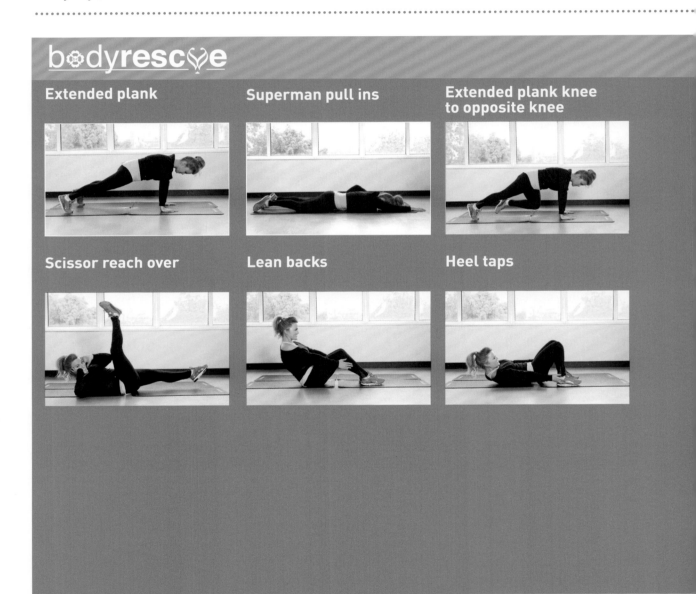

bodyrescue

| Extended plank | Superman pull ins | Extended plank knee to opposite knee |

| Scissor reach over | Lean backs | Heel taps |

Extended plank

Kneel on the floor. Straighten your arms, step your right leg back straight and then your left leg straight and hold that position. Focus on pulling your stomach muscles in and breathing evenly.

Superman pull ins

Lie on your front, stretch your arms out in front of you. Raise your right arm and your left leg 2 inches off the floor, reaching as far as you can. As you do this, pull your stomach in, breathing out. Lower down and breathe in. Repeat the other side.

Extended plank knee to opposite knee

Position as above, take your right knee towards your left knee, keeping your hips completely still, shoulders down your back. Take your right foot back and repeat to the other side. Make sure your hips stay still.

Scissor reach over

Lie on your back, take your legs in the air. Lower your left leg down about 10 inches. Take your hands either side of your head, and lift your head and shoulders off the floor. Take your left elbow towards the right leg, breathing out. Then take the left leg up towards you and lower the right leg down, at the same time as taking the right elbow to the left leg.

Lean backs

Sit on the floor, with your knees bent and feet on the floor. Take yours hands by the side of your legs and lean back, breathing out. Breathe in to come up.

Heel taps

Lie on your back, place the feet on the floor and lift the head and shoulders. Take your hands either side of the legs and, keeping your head looking towards your legs, stretch your right hand to your right foot, tapping the heel. Breathe out as you do this. Come back to the centre and breathe in. Breathe out and take your left hand to your left heel. And repeat.

15: Interval training 2

Once a week (from week 8-12)

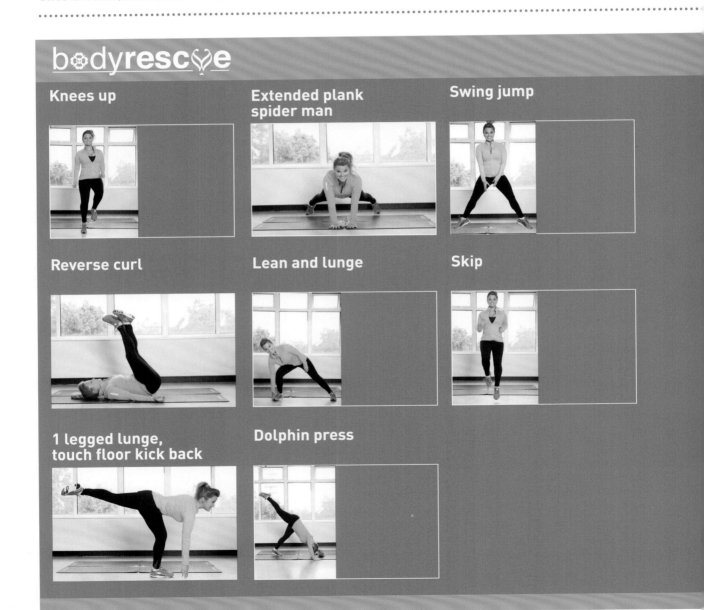

16: Explanation of moves

Knees up

In a standing position, take your right knee up as high as you can, and alternate knees. For more impact take both feet off the floor at the same time so you are running on the spot with high knees.

Extended plank spider man

Take the position of extended plank, but have your hands narrow, nearly touching, and open your legs wide. Now take your arms wide and your legs narrow as you walk to the right with your arms and legs. Keep moving in this direction, in this way. And then come back to the left.

Swing jump

In a standing position, take your legs wide with your feet turned out. Arms in the air, now bend your knees and take your arms through your legs in a fast motion, looking up and keeping your back flat. As you come up swing your arms in the air and jump.

Reverse curl

Lie on your back. Lift your legs in the air. Raise your bottom and lower back off the floor, and then back down again. Don't use your hands on the floor to help you, and don't push into your head. Lower down as gently as you can.

Lean and lunge

In a standing position, take your legs wide with your feet facing forwards. Bend at the knee and take your right hand to your right ankle, so straightening your left leg. Keep your head looking up and your back straight. Come back up to a standing position, and then lean to the left side, touching your left ankle. Repeat.

Skip

If you have a skipping rope, jump or run on the spot whilst skipping. If you do not have a rope then just jog or jump on the spot without one.

1 legged lunge, touch floor kick back

Take your right foot off the floor, and squat down with your left leg, touching your left hand to the floor, keeping your right foot just 2 inches off the floor. As you come up, extend the right leg behind you, straighten your leg and stretch your arm in front of you, repeat going down and up. Do right and left.

Dolphin press

In a downward dog position, take your right leg in the air, and press down towards the floor, elbows in, pushing chest to the floor and then back up again, keeping leg up all the time, repeat. Do right and left.

17: Resistance workout 2

Once a week (from Weeks 8-12)

bodyrescue

Spider man press ups
x 8 x 2

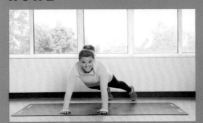

Plié jumps
x12 x 2

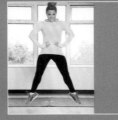

Tricep dips with leg in the air and hold x 15 x 2

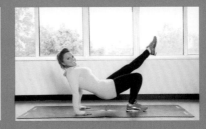

Alternate lunge jump
x16 x 2

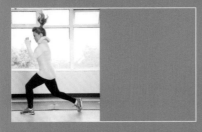

Mountain climbers
x20 x 2

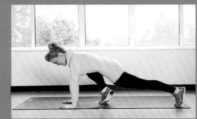

Side lunge jump
x16 x 2

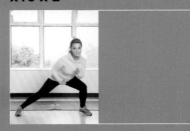

18: Explanation of moves

Spider man press ups

Same thing as extended plank spider man, except after moving 4 times to the right you press down, bending at the elbow, chest towards the floor, then 4 times to the left etc.

Plié jumps

Take your legs apart wide, and turn your toes out. Keep your back straight and bend the legs low. As you come up jump and reach up, then back down again and repeat.

Tricep dips with leg in the air and hold

Same position as tricep dips, but this time extending the right leg in the air as you bend from the elbow; repeat.

Alternate lunge jump

Lunge position, bend the knees. As you come up jump and change the legs over. Repeat.

Mountain climbers

Kneel and take your hands on the floor. Take your right knee into your chest, and your left leg straight. Alternate, making a fast motion one in one back.

Side lunge jump

The same as a lean and lunge, but this time adding a jump to each side position.

19: Stretch

(from weeks 2-12) **with resistance, cardio and Interval training.**

Perform at the end of the workout for 10 minutes- spend 10 seconds on each stretch.

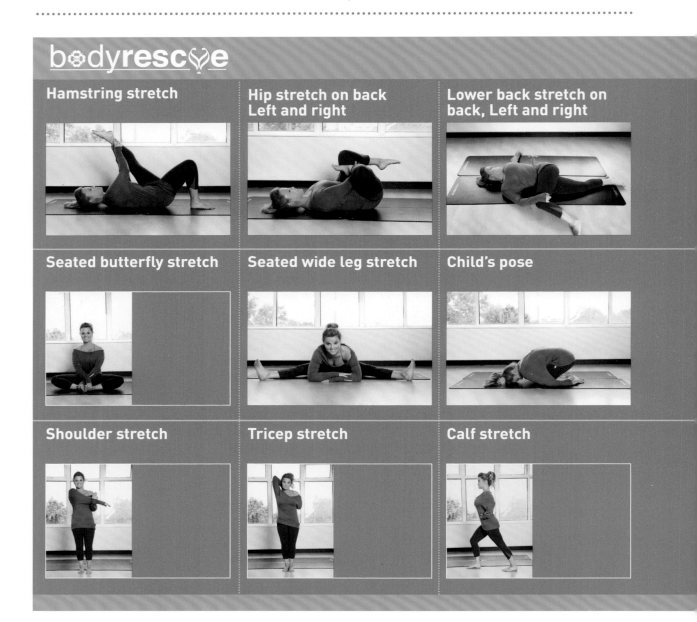

bodyrescue

Hamstring stretch	Hip stretch on back Left and right	Lower back stretch on back, Left and right
Seated butterfly stretch	Seated wide leg stretch	Child's pose
Shoulder stretch	Tricep stretch	Calf stretch

Hamstring stretch on back

Lie on your back, raise your right leg in the air, left knee bent with foot on the floor. Pull that right leg towards you with your hands behind the right leg. Do right and left. Hold for 10 seconds.

Forward bend

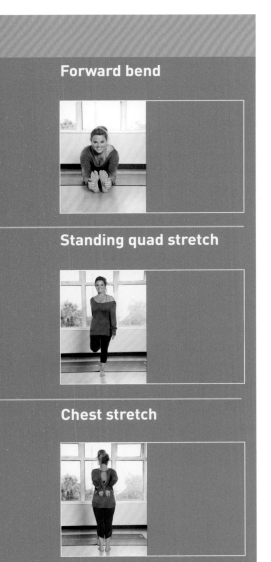

Standing quad stretch

Chest stretch

Hip stretch on back

In the same position, take your right foot on your left thigh, and place your hands behind your left leg. Keep your head on the floor. Raise your left foot of the floor, bringing the leg towards you.

Forward bend

In a seated position, straighten your legs in front of you, together. Reach to your feet.
Hold for 10 seconds.

Seated butterfly

In seated position, take your feet together, knees out to the side and try and push the knees to the floor. Hold for 10 seconds.

Seated wide leg

Take your legs wide and lean forwards, towards the floor.
Hold for 20 seconds.

Child's pose

From a kneeling position, take your head on the floor in front of you. Take your hands round towards the feet, hold the ankles if you can. You can make this easier by widening the legs.
Hold 10 seconds.

Standing quad stretch

Stand and hold onto your right foot, with your right hand, knee touching the other knee. Hold 10 seconds. Repeat other side

Shoulder stretch

Take your right arm towards your left shoulder, straight. Place your left hand on your right upper arm, pulling it towards you closer. Hold for 10 seconds. Repeat other side.

Lower back stretch

Hug your right knee towards you, and straighten the left leg on the floor. Take your right arm out to the side and roll the hip to the left. Hold for 10 seconds. Repeat both sides.

Tricep stretch

Take your right arm up in the air. Place the right hand on the back of the neck, bending at the elbow. Reach your left arm up the back to find your right hand and hold them together if you can. If you cannot reach them together, a good tip is to hold on to a sock with the upper hand, let it dangle and grab it with the lower hand. Then walk the hands together. Hold for 10 seconds. Do right and left.

Calf stretch

Place your hands on the wall. Take your right leg back and push through the heel, feeling a deep calf stretch, bending the left leg too. Hold for 10 seconds and repeat other side.

Chest stretch

Place your hands in the arch of your back, palms down. Squeeze the elbows in towards each other. If you can, get someone else to gently push your elbows together. This feels amazing, as most of the day we are rounded in the back, driving, texting, typing etc... Hold for 20 seconds.

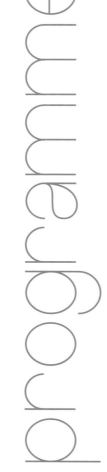

The Body Rescue exercise programme

20: Weeks 1- 12

Week 1

Mindset - programming – every day
Visualise yourself as how you want to be and write down your goals.
Do your vision board (see ch 1)

Abdominals
30 Reverse curls
10 Supermans
6 Lean back and twist
5 Bridge
50 Pullins
As you are in the first week of your detox you may be feeling tired, so all I want you to do this week are your abdominals exercises.

Week 2

Mindset - visualise every day

Exercise

3 cardio workouts a week
- can be cycling, swimming, fast walking, jogging, gym cardio machines (treadmill, rower, stepper, cross trainer) **30-45mins.**

Abdominals - every day
50 Reverse curls
10 Supermans
10 Lean back and twist
10 Bridge
60 Pullins

Week 3

Mindset - visualise every day
Visualise goals every day and gratitude diary.

Exercise

3 cardio workouts a week

1 Resistance training

1 Interval training

Abdominals - every day
50 reverse curls
12 Supermans
10 Lean back and twist
10 Bridge
70 Pullins

Week 4

Mindset - visualise - every day

Exercise

3 cardio workouts a week

- can be cycling, swimming, fast walking, jogging, gym cardio machines (treadmill, rower, stepper, cross trainer) **30-45mins.**

1 Yoga

Abdominals - every day

60 Reverse curls
16 Supermans
16 Lean back and twist
15 Bridge
80 Pullins

1 Resistance training once a week

Week 5

Mindset - visualise every day

Exercise

3 cardio workouts a week

- can be cycling, swimming, fast walking, jogging, gym cardio machines (treadmill, rower, stepper, cross trainer) **30-45mins.**

1 Interval training

1 Yoga

Abdominals every day

70 Reverse curls
20 Supermans
20 Lean back and twist
20 Bridge
90 Pullins

1 Resistance training once a week

Week 6

Mindset- visualise every day
Exercise

3 cardio workouts a week

- can be cycling, swimming, fast walking, jogging, gym cardio machines (treadmill, rower, stepper, cross trainer) **30-45mins.**

1 Interval training

1 Yoga

Abdominals- every day

100 Reverse curls
20 Supermans

20 Lean back and twist
20 Bridge
100 Pullins

Resistance training once a week

Week 7

Mindset- visualise every day

Exercise

3 cardio workouts a week

- can be cycling, swimming, fast walking, jogging, gym cardio machines (treadmill, rower, stepper, cross trainer) **30-45mins.**

1 Interval training

1 Yoga

1 Abdominals every day

100 Reverse curls
26 Supermans
26 Lean back and twist
20 Bridge
100 Pullins

1 Resistance training once a week

Week 8

Mindset- visualise every day

Exercise

3 cardio workouts a week

- can be cycling, swimming, fast walking, jogging, gym cardio machines (treadmill, rower, stepper, cross trainer) **30-45mins.**

2 Interval training

1 Yoga

Abdominals every day

30 seconds Extended plank
50 Superman pull ins
10 Extended plank knee to opposite knee
50 Scissor sit up
10 Lean backs
50 Heel taps

2 Resistance training once a week

Week 9

Mindset- visualise every day

Exercise

3 cardio workouts a week

- can be cycling, swimming, fast walking, jogging,

gym cardio machines (treadmill, rower, stepper, cross trainer) **30-45mins.**

2 Interval training

1 Yoga

Abdominals every day

40 seconds Extended plank
60 Superman pull ins
14 Extended plank knee to opposite knee
60 Scissor sit up
14 Lean backs
60 Heel taps

2 Resistance training once a week

Week 10

Mindset- visualise every day

Exercise

3 cardio workouts a week- can be cycling, swimming, fast walking, jogging, gym cardio machines (treadmill, rower, stepper, cross trainer) **30-45mins.**

2 Interval training

1 Yoga

Abdominals every day
50 seconds Extended plank
70 Superman pull ins
16 Extended plank knee to opposite knee
70 Scissor sit up
16 Lean backs
70 Heel taps

2 Resistance training once a week.

Week 11

Mindset- visualise every day

Exercise

3 cardio workouts a week
- can be cycling, swimming, fast walking, jogging, gym cardio machines (treadmill, rower, stepper, cross trainer) **30-45mins.**

2 Interval training

1 Yoga

Abdominals every day
60 seconds Extended plank
80 Superman pull ins
18 Extended plank knee to opposite knee
80 Scissor sit up

18 Lean backs
80 Heel taps

2 Resistance training once a week.

Week 12

Mindset- visualise every day

Exercise

3 cardio workouts a week
- can be cycling, swimming, fast walking, jogging, gym cardio machines (treadmill, rower, stepper, cross trainer) **30-45mins.**

2 Interval training

1 Yoga

Abdominals every day
70 seconds Extended plank
80 Superman pull ins
20 Extended plank knee to opposite knee
90 Scissor sit up
20 Lean backs
80 Heel taps

2 Resistance training once a week

Maintenance from week 13 onwards

Mindset- visualise every day

Exercise

3 cardio workouts a week
- can be cycling, swimming, fast walking, jogging, gym cardio machines (treadmill, rower, stepper, cross trainer) **30-45mins.**

1 Interval training

1 Yoga

Abdominals every day
70 seconds Extended plank
80 Superman pull ins
20 Extended plank knee to opposite knee
90 Scissor sit up
20 Lean backs
80 Heel taps

Resistance training once a week

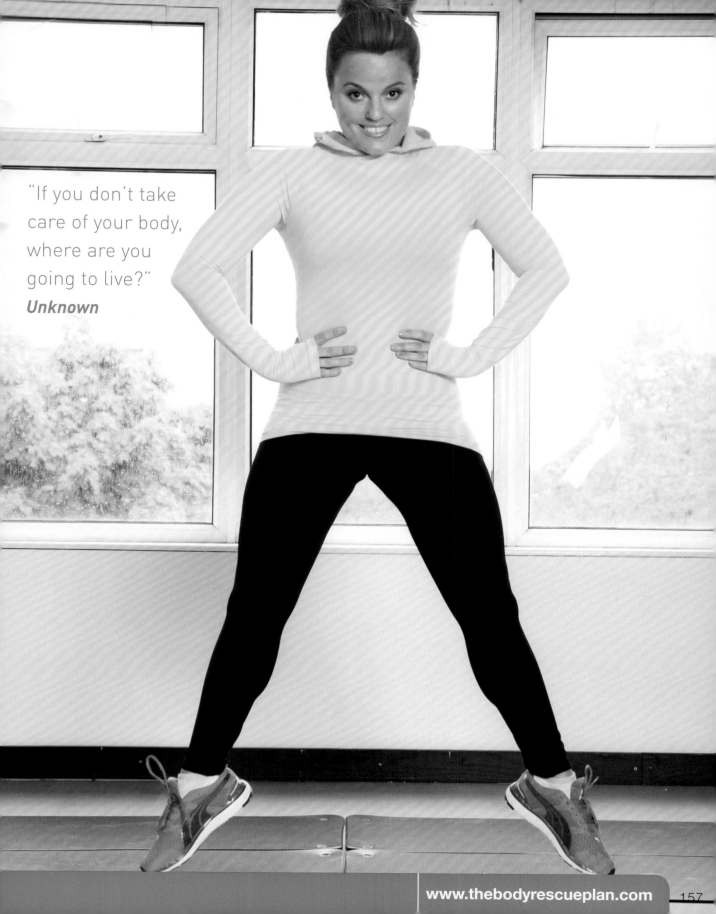

"If you don't take care of your body, where are you going to live?"
Unknown

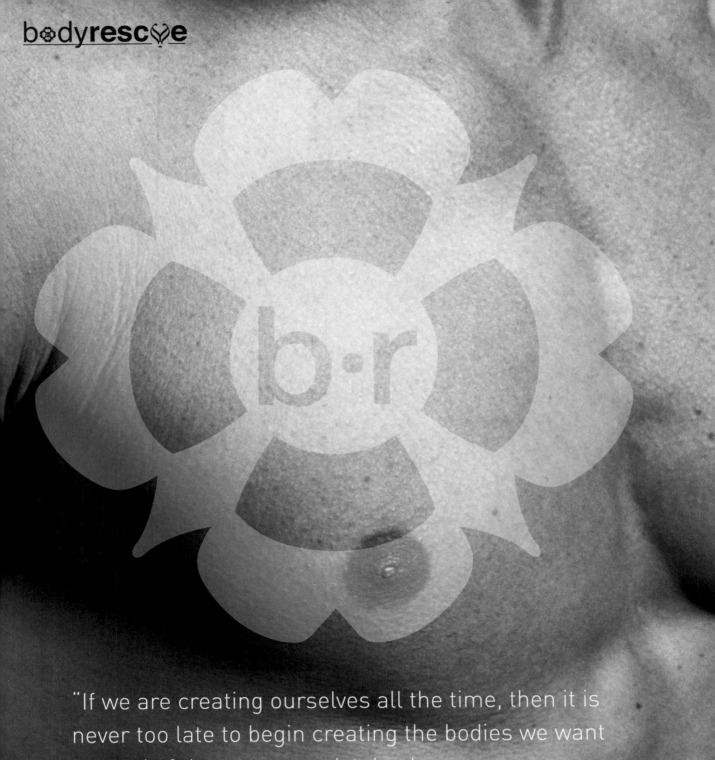

bodyrescue

"If we are creating ourselves all the time, then it is never too late to begin creating the bodies we want instead of the ones we mistakenly assume we are stuck with."
Deepak Chopra link

Chapter 9
Yoga and meditation

01: Why Yoga?
02: Free Meditation CD download
03: The Body Rescue Yoga Chart
04: Explanation of the Yoga postures

Yoga and meditation Introduction

There are many reasons I ask my clients to practise yoga, but in terms of weight loss it is very beneficial.

A stressed body and mind will create a body that holds onto fat, and a mind that is far more likely to reach for the biscuit tin and lack in willpower.

A controlled body and mind will make rational decisions to make their body feel even more amazing, and create a beautiful eco system in their body so that their hormones, organs cells and every part of them works efficiently, and that is where yoga comes in.

01: Why Yoga?

Yoga asanas (postures) cleanse our glands and organs, helping them to produce a healing chemical balance for detoxification and a calming effect. Yoga improves circulation, sending invigorating oxygen to your brain and all your muscles. The stretching and strengthening movements allow the body to tone and increase flexibility.

Yoga increases the body's chi energy, which allows one to gain an inner strength. The circulation and cardiovascular system is also improved by improving blood flow to that area of the body.

Yoga is combined with complete relaxation and meditation techniques that show you how to access the strength and power of your inner self, for a support system that maintains your will and mental strength.

Yoga focusses on deep invigorating breathing techniques which bring large amounts of fresh oxygen to the brain and other parts of the body. Yoga reaches parts of the body you perhaps didn't know existed.

Yoga helps raise the feel good chemicals in our body which in turn helps eliminate the physiological manifestations of stress – which could harbour in aches in the neck, back head, or stress in the stomach and chest, to name but a few. The fluid movements act as a wonderful remedy for aching limbs

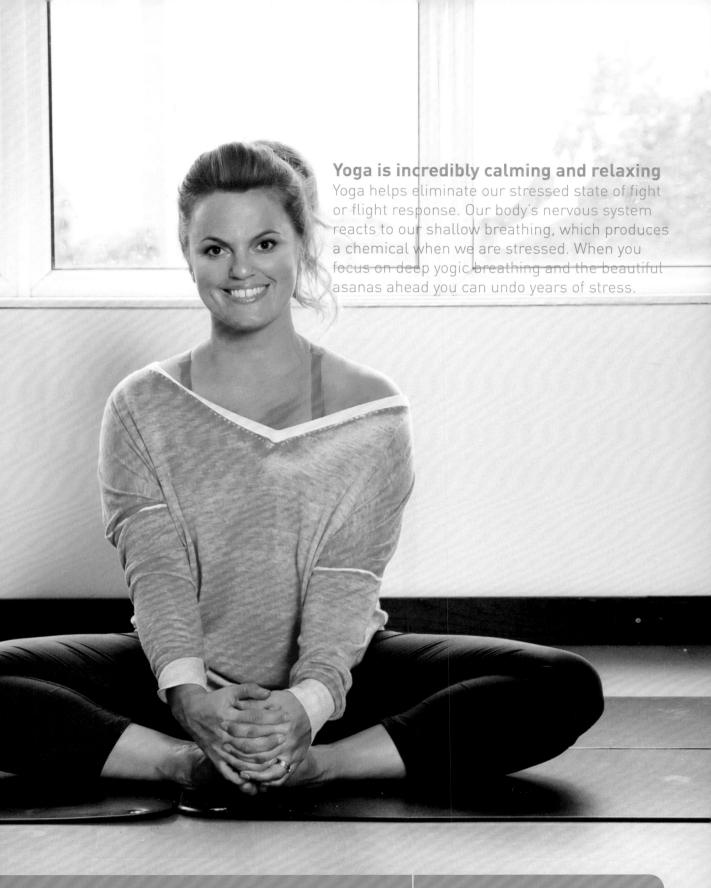

Yoga is incredibly calming and relaxing
Yoga helps eliminate our stressed state of fight or flight response. Our body's nervous system reacts to our shallow breathing, which produces a chemical when we are stressed. When you focus on deep yogic breathing and the beautiful asanas ahead you can undo years of stress.

02: Download your FREE Meditation CD now!

To download your FREE meditation CD **please go to the following link**
http://www.thebodyrescueplan.com/meditation-audio-request/
and enter the code TBRP1

Please note you cannot download directly onto a phone or I pad. To get the meditations onto your phone or iPad you can download to your computer onto I tunes and then this can upload to your phone or I pad.

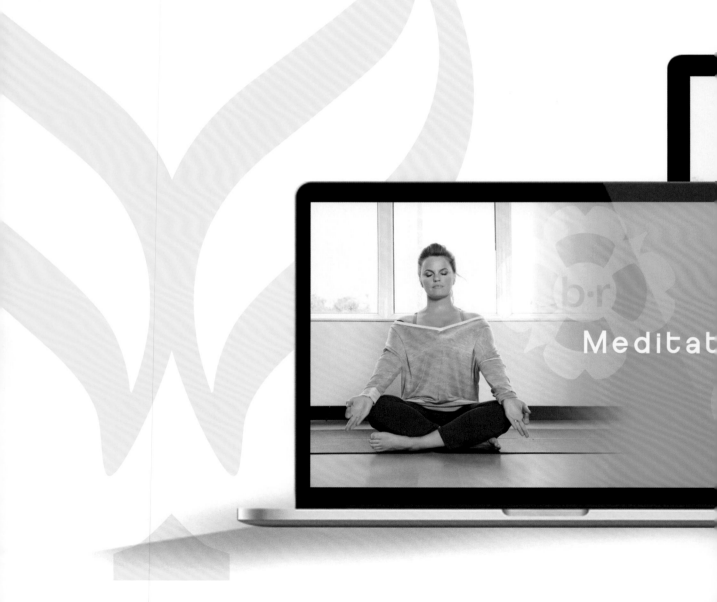

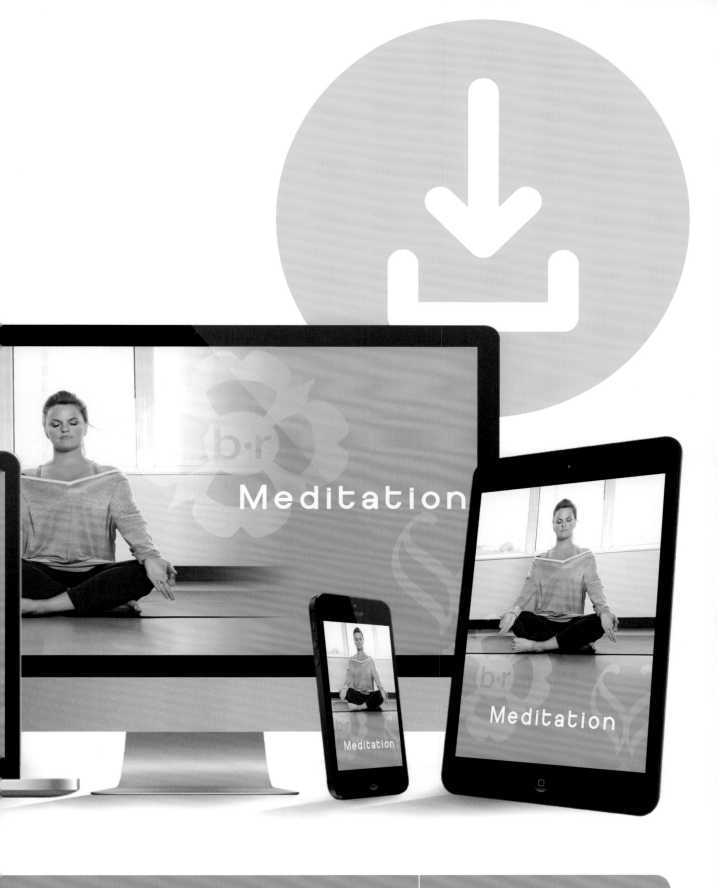

03: The Body Rescue
Yoga Chart

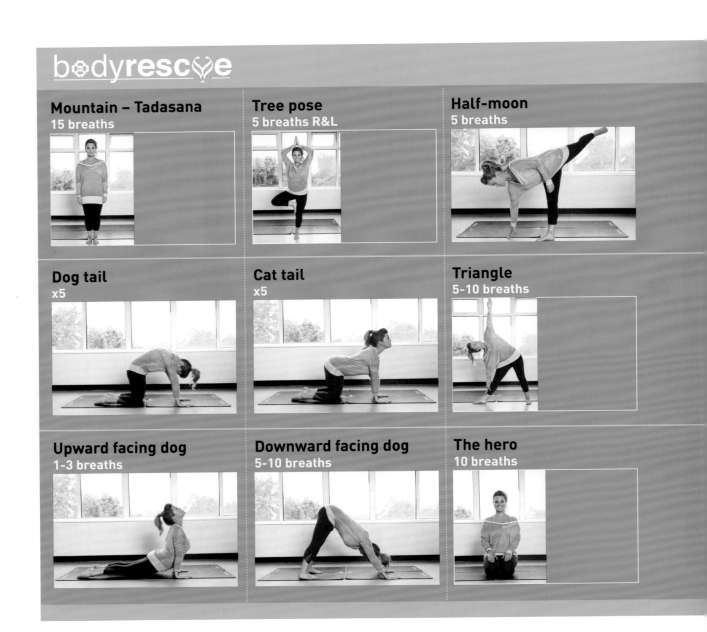

bodyrescue

Mountain – Tadasana
15 breaths

Tree pose
5 breaths R&L

Half-moon
5 breaths

Dog tail
x5

Cat tail
x5

Triangle
5-10 breaths

Upward facing dog
1-3 breaths

Downward facing dog
5-10 breaths

The hero
10 breaths

"Reach for the thoughts that feel better – and watch what happens."

Christianne Wolff

The following postures should be performed after warming up for 10 minutes – you can do 5 sun salutations to warm up or use the warm up sequence in the exercise section. Please hold each posture for the allocated breaths in the chart below, and make sure your IN breath is the same speed as your OUT breath. Ground yourself and BREATHE.

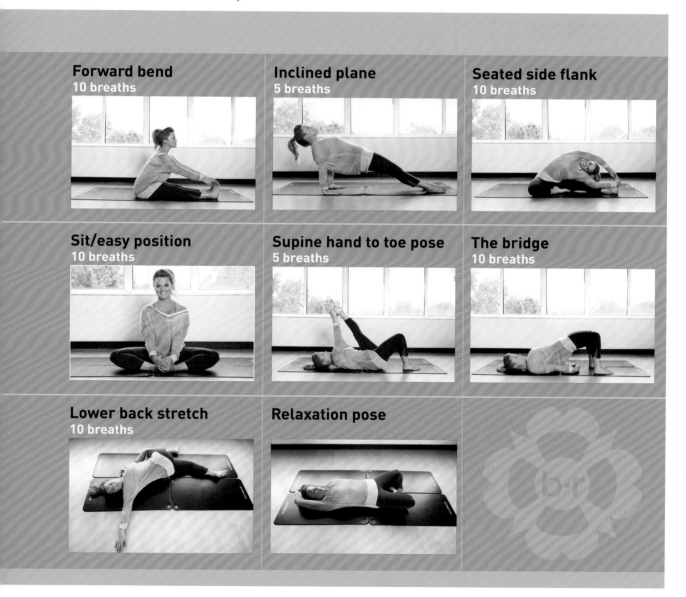

Forward bend
10 breaths

Inclined plane
5 breaths

Seated side flank
10 breaths

Sit/easy position
10 breaths

Supine hand to toe pose
5 breaths

The bridge
10 breaths

Lower back stretch
10 breaths

Relaxation pose

04: Explanation of the yoga postures

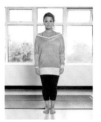

Mountain – Tadasana

Improves posture, balance and self-awareness.

Stand with your feet hip distance apart and focus on your breathing, shoulders down the back, knees relaxed, belly pulled in, and lift head tall. Breathe evenly in and out, and focus on your breath relaxing you. Take 15 breaths.

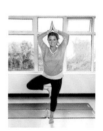

Tree pose – vrikshasana

Aids balance, focus, and concentration and is strengthening to the ankles and knees.

Focus your eyes on one point in front of you and place your right foot on your left inner thigh, if you find your foot is slipping try your foot on bare skin. Repeat other side. 5 breaths each side, or as long as you can.

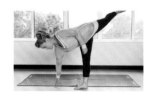

Half-moon posture

Increases flexibility in the groin, strengthens the arms, lengthens the hamstrings.

From a standing position, take your right hand to your right foot, trying to keep your legs straight. Raise your left leg off the floor, straightening that leg up towards the sky. Hold for 5 breaths and do the other side.

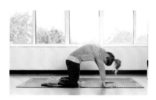

Dog tail

mobilises the spine.

On all fours, round your back so you feel like you are rounding over a ball.

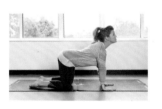

Cat tail

Mobilises the spine and opens up the chest and shoulders.

From Dog tail, arch your back so that you are looking up to the sky, repeat these together for 1 breath each x 5

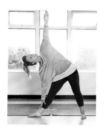

Triangle

Stand with your feet apart, if you take your arms out wide and look at where your wrists are they should be in line with your ankles. Now turn your left foot in and your right foot out, and keeping your hips forwards, lean to the right so your right hand touches your shin or ankle (keep your legs straight). Your left hand wants to face up to the sky and your gaze is to your left hand. Hold for 5-10 breaths and repeat the other side. When you come out of the posture breathe in.

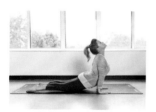

Upward facing dog – urdvha mukha svanasana

Blood moves into the pelvic region, increasing health and vitality. People with back problems can gain relief by practising it.

From a lying position on your front, take your hands under your shoulders, straighten your arms and lift your thighs off the floor at the same time. Pulling the shoulders down the back, keeping the tops of the feet on the floor. Do not take your neck right back. If this is too deep a stretch for you, then go to cobra, keeping legs on the ground and bending at

the elbows.
Hold for 1-3 breaths.

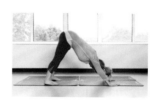

Downward facing dog – adho mukha svanasana

Builds strength, flexibility and awareness, and all round strengthening posture and stretches the spine and hamstrings.

From a standing position take your hands to the floor, step your feet back behind you so that your bottom is in the air, creating a triangle shape. Relax your head, push your chest into the floor, pull up through the thighs and push down through the heels. Hold for 5-10 breaths. If you are not flexible enough to hold the posture, try bending your knees a little to enable your back to be straight, and then in turn try straightening your legs and round your back.

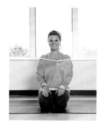

The hero–virasana

Is excellent for meditation; it softens the hips, knees and ankles.

Kneel on the floor with your buttocks placed on the heels and your hands on your knees. Hold for 10 breaths.

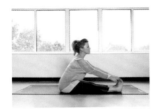

Forward bend-
Lengthening hamstrings and opening up the back.

In a seated position, straighten your legs, place your hands under the buttocks and pull them back behind you. Then take your hands towards your feet, keeping your back straight and your chest lifted. Hold for 10 breaths.

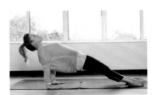

Inclined plane – purvottanasana
Tones and strengthens the whole body (especially core body strength) and opens the chest.

Sit on the floor and straighten your legs. Place your hands by your hips with your fingers forward. Lift your hips off the floor. Hold for 5 breaths.

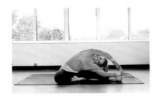

Seated side flank – parsvakonasana
Strengthens and stretches the legs, knees, and ankles. Stretches the groin, spine, chest and lungs, and shoulders. Stimulates abdominal organs. Improves digestion and aids elimination.

Sit with your right knee bent and your right foot on your left inner thigh.

Take your left hand out towards the left leg, then turn it on its back and then round again, then grab the base of the foot. Reach your right arm over towards the left hand and open the chest out.
Breathe 10. Repeat other side.

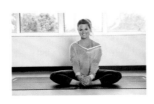

Sit/easy position – sukhasana
A starting position that helps focus awareness on breathing and the body; helps strengthen lower back and open the groin and hips.

Sit with your feet together and knees out to the side. Back straight. Breathe for 10.

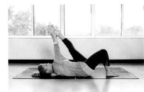

Supine hand to toe pose – hasta padangustasana
A good hamstring stretch, opens the hips and realigns the spine.

Lie on your back, straighten both of your legs and raise your left leg towards your face; lifting your head and shoulders off the floor, take your hands behind your left thigh and pull towards you. Hold for 10 breaths. Repeat other side.

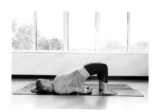

The bridge – Sethu Bandhasa

Strengthens and stretches the lower back and abdominal muscles; opens the chest.

Lie on your back, with your knees bent and your feet on the floor. Lift your hips off the floor and place your hands on the floor and hold for 10 breaths.

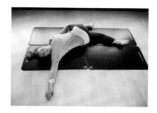

Lower back stretch

Hug your right knee towards you, and straighten the left leg on the floor. Take your right arm out to the side and roll the hip to the left. Hold for 10 breaths. Repeat both sides.

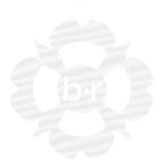

04: When to do your yoga practice?

It is best to practice yoga on an empty stomach, after at least an hour and a half without food; you can go so much deeper into the postures and they are a lot more enjoyable. You may do your yoga practice after a cardio session or resistance training session, or just on its own.

05: What do I wear for yoga?

I would really recommend Bamboo clothing; they are beautifully natural garments, and really comfortable

06: Yoga relaxation exercise for stress

Try the following tense-relax exercise as you lie in the corpse pose:

1. As you inhale through your nose, tighten the muscles in your knees, calves, ankles, feet, and toes. Hold the tension, then relax and exhale.

2. Inhale, tensing all of these parts as well as your abdomen, pelvis, hips, and thighs. Hold them taut, then relax and exhale.

3. Tense the muscles in your neck, shoulders, arms, elbows, waist, hands, fingers, and chest, as well as the muscles in your trunk and legs. Hold the tension, then relax and exhale.

4. Finally, starting with your scalp, face, and head, tense all of your body muscles. Hold the tension, then relax and exhale. Feel how all of the tension has melted away from your body.

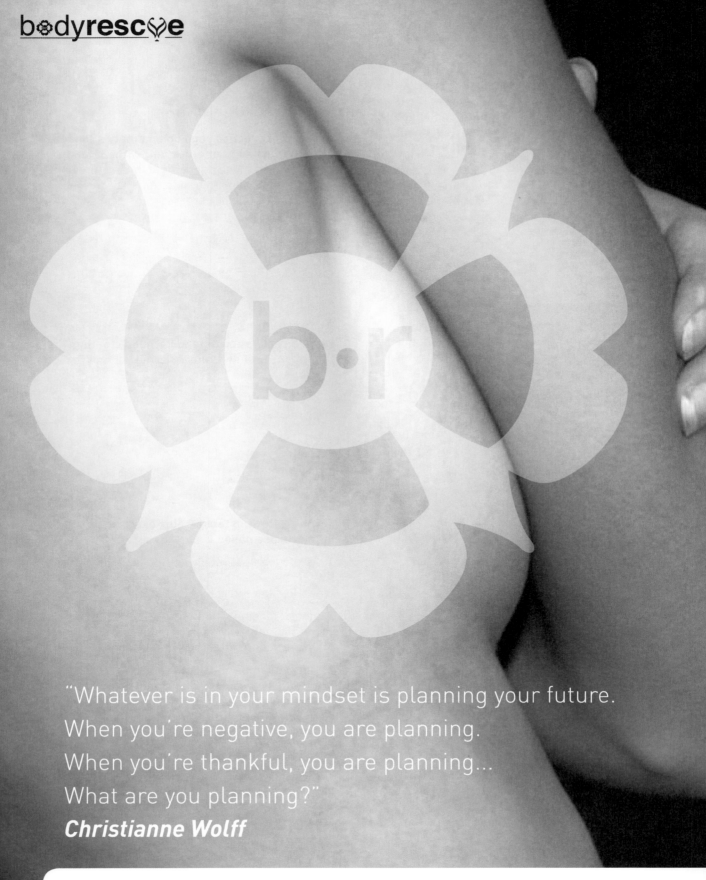

"Whatever is in your mindset is planning your future.
When you're negative, you are planning.
When you're thankful, you are planning...
What are you planning?"
Christianne Wolff

Chapter 10
Your Body Rescue Weekly Plan

Weeks 1 -13

Your Body Rescue
Weekly Plan

To make it easier for you to see how your weeks should look, in this chapter I have created a series of weekly plans that summarise the complete 13 weeks of the Body Resue plan.

The Body Rescue Weekly Plan is a simple guided overview, and a daily diary for you to monitor your progress.

Listed at the top of each Weekly Plan are my suggestions that give examples of the type activity and and diet you can plan for each day.

At the lower end of each Weekly Plan are listed the mindset/meditation, exercise and eating for each week, with blank spaces for you to enter your actions and plans completed for each day.

- **Put in the Weekly Plan diary** - **what you are going to eat and when you are going to prepare it.**
- **Put in the Weekly Plan diary** - **when you will exercise and stick to it!**

Preparation is the KEY!

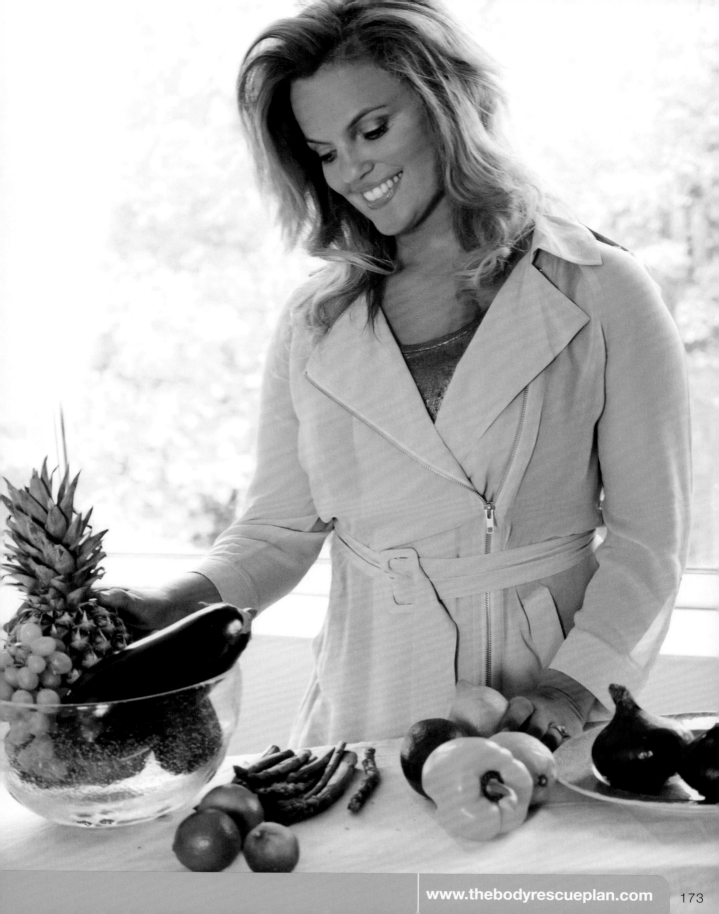

bodyrescue

Week 1	Monday	Tuesday	Wednesday
	Meditation Visualise goals **Mindset** Do vision board	**Meditation** Fears **Mindset** Look at vision board	**Meditation** Guilt **Mindset** Look at vision board
	Abs 30 Reverse curls; 10 Supermans; 6 Lean back and twist; 5 Bridge; 50 Pullins	**Abs** 30 Reverse curls; 10 Supermans; 6 Lean back and twist; 5 Bridge; 50 Pullins	**Abs** 30 Reverse curls; 10 Supermans; 6 Lean back and twist; 5 Bridge; 50 Pullins
	Breakfast Psyllium husks, spirulina, aloe vera. Hot water and lemon. Apple, carrot and ginger juice	**Breakfast** Psyllium husks, spirulina, aloe vera. Hot water and lemon. Berry smoothie with milled flaxseeds.	**Breakfast** Psyllium husks, spirulina, aloe vera. Hot water and lemon. Steamed plums.
	Snack Cashew nuts and raisins **Lunch** Sweet potato with roasted veg. **Snack** Psyllium husks, spirulina, Nakd bar **Supper** Sea bream and vegetables	**Snack** Nuts and seeds **Lunch** Corn on the cob with ratatouille **Snack** Psyllium husks, spirulina, Nakd bar. **Supper** Chicken and vegetables	**Snack** Nuts and seeds **Lunch** Prawn salad **Snack** Psyllium husks, spirulina Nakd bar **Supper** Vegetable curry
	Gratitude diary	**Gratitude diary**	**Gratitude diary**

Your Body Rescue Weekly Plan

Weekly Plan diary

Meditation/Mindset Visualise goals and do vision board. **Gratitude diary**			
Exercise Just abs 30 Reverse curls			
10 Supermans			
6 Lean back and twist			
5 Bridge			
50 Pullins			
Eating **Detox wk 1** Fruit, veg, fish, white meat, fistful nuts, seeds and dried fruit			

Thursday	Friday	Saturday	Sunday
Meditation Self sabotage **Mindset** **Look at vision board**	**Meditation** Greed **Mindset** **Look at vision board**	**Meditation** Visualise goals **Mindset** **Do vision board**	**Day off exercise**
Abs 30 Reverse curls;10 Supermans; 6 Lean back and twist; 5 Bridge; 50 Pullins	**Abs** 30 Reverse curls; 10 Supermans; 6 Lean back and twist; 5 Bridge; 50 Pullins	**Abs** 30 Reverse curls;10 Supermans; 6 Lean back and twist; 5 Bridge; 50 Pullins	**Breakfast** Psyllium husks, spirulina. Hot water and lemon. Orange, apple, carrot and grapefruit juice.
Breakfast Psyllium husks, spirulina, aloe vera. Hot water and lemon. Pineapple and melon smoothy.	**Breakfast** Psyllium husks, spirulina. Hot water and lemon.Carrot, apple, strawberry cabbage juice.	**Breakfast** Psyllium husks, spirulina, aloe vera. Hot water and lemon. Apple, carrot and ginger juice.	**Snack** Nuts and seeds **Lunch** Vegetable omelette **Snack** Psyllium husks, spirulina Nakd bar
Snack Nuts and seeds **Lunch** Salad Niçoise **Snack** Psyllium husks, spirulina Nakd bar **Supper** Chilli butternut squash	**Snack** Nuts and seeds **Lunch** Sweet potato salad **Snack** Psyllium husks, spirulina Nakd bar **Supper** Tuna frittata	**Snack** Cashew nuts and raisins **Lunch** Sweet potato with roasted veg. **Snack** Psyllium husks, spirulina, Nakd bar **Supper** Sea bream and vegetables	**Supper** Salmon salad
Gratitude diary	**Gratitude diary**	**Gratitude diary**	**Gratitude diary**

bodyrescᴏe

Your Body Rescue Weekly Plan

Week 2	Monday	Tuesday	Wednesday
	Meditation Visualise goals **Mindset** Make focus wheel **Exercise** Abs 50 Reverse curls 10 Superman 10 Lean back and twist 10 Bridge 60 Pullins Bike ride 30 mins **Breakfast** Psyllium husks, spirulina, aloe vera. Hot water and lemon. Yogurt and bananas. **Snack** Cashew nuts and raisins **Lunch** Rice salad. **Snack** Psyllium husks, spirulina, Nakd bar **Supper** Salmon and vegetables **Gratitude diary**	**Meditation** Visualise goals **Exercise** Abs 50 Reverse curls 10 Superman 10 Lean back and twist 10 Bridge 60 Pullins **Gratitude diary**	**Meditation** Stress **Exercise** Abs 50 reverse curls 10 Superman 10 Lean back and twist 10 Bridge 60 Pullins Swim 30 mins **Gratitude diary**

Weekly Plan diary

Meditation Goals every day **Gratitude diary**			
Exercise 50 Reverse curls			
10 Supermans			
10 Lean back and twist			
10 Bridge			
60 Pullins			
2-3 cardio workouts a week			
Eating **Detox wk2** As above plus plain yogurt, banana, and fistful of carbs in oats, potatoes, rice, pasta, couscous.			

Thursday	Friday	Saturday	Sunday
Meditation Greed	**Meditation** Fear	**Meditation** Visualise goals	**Day off exercise**
Exercise Abs 50 Reverse curls 10 Superman 10 Lean back and twist 10 Bridge 60 Pullins	**Exercise** Abs 50 Reverse curls 10 Superman 10 Lean back and twist 10 Bridge 60 Pullins	**Exercise** Abs 50 Reverse curls 10 Superman 10 Lean back and twist 10 Bridge 60 Pullins Fast walk 30 mins	
Gratitude diary	**Gratitude diary**	**Gratitude diary**	

bodyrescue

bodyrescue

Week 3

Your Body Rescue Weekly Plan

	Monday	**Tuesday**	**Wednesday**
Meditation	Visualise goals	Fears	Guilt
Exercise	Abs 50 Reverse curls 12 Supermans 10 Lean back and twist 10 Bridge 70 Pullins Bike Ride 30 mins	Abs 50 Reverse curls 12 Supermans 10 Lean back and twist 10 Bridge 70 Pullins Resistance training	Abs 50 Reverse curls 12 Supermans 10 Lean back and twist 10 Bridge 70 Pullins Swim 30 mins
	Breakfast Psyllium husks, spirulina, aloe vera. Hot water and lemon. Porridge with banana. **Snack** Cashew nuts and raisins **Lunch** Feta cheese salad. **Snack** Psyllium husks, spirulina, Nakd bar. **Supper** Lentil curry.	**Gratitude diary**	**Gratitude diary**
	Gratitude diary		

Weekly Plan diary

Meditation Goals every day **Gratitude diary**			
Exercise 2-3 cardio workouts a week			
1 Resistance training			
1 Interval training			
50 Reverse curls			
12 Supermans			
10 Lean back and twist			
10 Bridge			
70 Pullins			
Eating As above plus 1 matchbox size of cheese, or 2 matchbox size of goats' cheese a day. As much pulses as you like (lentils, beans, chickpeas etc.) 2.5 litres of water.			

Thursday	Friday	Saturday	Sunday
Meditation Sabotage	**Meditation** Stress	**Meditation** Visualise goals	**Day off exercise**
Exercise Abs 50 Reverse curls 12 Supermans 10 Lean back and twist 10 Bridge 70 Pullins Interval training	**Exercise** Abs 50 Reverse curls 12 Supermans 10 Lean back and twist 10 Bridge 70 Pullins Jog 30 mins	**Exercise** Abs 50 Reverse curls; 12 Supermans 10 Lean back and twist 10 Bridge 70 Pullins	
Gratitude diary	**Gratitude diary**	**Gratitude diary**	

bodyrescue

Your Body Rescue Weekly Plan

Week 4	Monday	Tuesday	Wednesday
Meditation	Visualise goals	Fears	Guilt
Exercise	Abs 60 Reverse curls 16 Supermans 16 Lean back and twist 15 Bridge 80 Pullins Bike Ride 30 mins	Abs 60 Reverse curls 16 Supermans 16 Lean back and twist 15 Bridge 80 Pullins Resistance training	Abs 60 Reverse curls 16 Supermans 16 Lean back and twist 15 Bridge 80 Pullins Swim 30 mins
	Breakfast Psyllium husks, spirulina, aloe vera. Hot water and lemon. Fruit Salad **Snack** Yogurt, milled flaxseeds and agave nectar. **Lunch** Jacket with cheese. **Snack** Psyllium husks, spirulina, Nakd bar. **Supper** Chickpea curry	Gratitude diary	Gratitude diary
	Gratitude diary		

Weekly Plan diary

	Monday	Tuesday	Wednesday
Meditation Goals every day **Gratitude diary**			
Exercise 1 Resistance training a week			
3 cardio workouts a week 30 - 45 mins			
1 Interval training			
60 Reverse curls			
16 Supermans			
16 Lean back and twist			
15 Bridge			
80 Pullins			
Yoga			
Eating As above plus 2 tbsps of agave nectar. Chocolate chips sugar free.			

Thursday	Friday	Saturday	Sunday
Meditation Sabotage	**Meditation** Stress	**Meditation** Visualise goals	**Day off exercise**
Exercise Abs 60 Reverse curls 16 Supermans 16 Lean back and twist 15 Bridge 80 Pullins Yoga	**Exercise** Abs 60 Reverse curls 16 Supermans 16 Lean back and twist 15 Bridge 80 Pullins Jog 30 mins	**Exercise** Abs 60 Reverse curls 16 Supermans 16 Lean back and twist 15 Bridge 80 Pullins seconds Interval training	
Gratitude diary	**Gratitude diary**	**Gratitude diary**	

bodyrescue

Week 5

	Monday	Tuesday	Wednesday
Meditation	Visualise goals	Fears	Guilt
Exercise	Abs 70 Reverse curls 20 Supermans 20 Lean back and twist 20 Bridge 90 Pullins Bike ride 30 mins	Abs 70 Reverse curls 20 Superman; 20 Lean back and twist 20 Bridge 90 Pullins Resistance training	Abs 70 Reverse curls 20 Superman; 20 Lean back and twist 20 Bridge 90 Pullins Swim 30 mins
	Breakfast Psyllium husks, spirulina, aloe vera. Hot water and lemon. Porridge with coconut milk, lime and agave nectar. **Snack** Yogurt, milled flaxseeds and agave nectar. **Lunch** Salmon ramen with noodles and soy sauce. **Snack** Psyllium husks, spirulina, Nakd bar. **Supper** Lentil salad.	**Gratitude diary**	**Gratitude diary**
	Gratitude diary		

Your Body Rescue Weekly Plan

Weekly Plan diary

Meditation Goals every day **Gratitude diary**			
Exercise 3 cardio workouts a week			
1 Interval training			
1 Resistance training			
Abs			
70 Reverse curls			
20 Supermans			
20 Lean back and twist			
20 Bridge			
90 Pullins			
Yoga			
Eating As above plus cornflour coconut milk soya sauce			

	Thursday	Friday	Saturday	Sunday
Meditation	Sabotage	Stress	Visualise goals	**Day off exercise**
Exercise	Abs	Abs	Abs	
	70 Reverse curls	70 Reverse curls	70 Reverse curls	
	20 Superman	20 Superman	20 Superman	
	20 Lean back and twist	20 Lean back and twist	20 Lean back and twist;	
	20 Bridge	20 Bridge	20 Bridge	
	90 Pullins	90 Pullins	90 Pullins	
	Yoga	Jog 30 mins	Interval training	
Gratitude diary				

bodyrescue

Week 6

	Monday	Tuesday	Wednesday
Meditation	Visualise goals	Fears	Guilt
Exercise	Abs 100 Reverse curls 20 Supermans 20 Lean back and twist 20 Bridge 100 Pullins Bike ride 30 mins	Abs 100 Reverse curls 20 Supermans 20 Lean back and twist 20 Bridge 100 Pullins Resistance training	Abs 100 Reverse curls; 20 Supermans 20 Lean back and twist 20 Bridge 100 Pullins Swim 30 mins
	Breakfast Psyllium husks, spirulina, aloe vera. Hot water and lemon. Fruit Salad **Snack** Yogurt, milled flaxseeds and agave nectar. **Lunch** Lentil soup. **Snack** Psyllium husks, spirulina, Nakd bar **Supper** Shepherd's pie	**Gratitude diary**	**Gratitude diary**
	Gratitude diary		

Your Body Rescue Weekly Plan

Weekly Plan diary

	Monday	Tuesday	Wednesday
Meditation Goals every day **Gratitude diary**			
Exercise 3 cardio workouts 30-45mins			
1 Interval training			
1 Resistance training			
100 Reverse curls			
20 Supermans			
20 Lean back and twist			
20 Bridge			
100 Pullins			
Yoga			
Eating Eating as above plus 1 glass rice milk 1 portion red meat a week			

Thursday	Friday	Saturday	Sunday
Meditation Sabotage	**Meditation** Stress	**Meditation** Visualise goals	**Day off exercise**
Exercise Abs 100 Reverse curls 20 Supermans 20 Lean back and twist 20 Bridge 100 Pullins Yoga	**Exercise** Abs 100 Reverse curls 20 Supermans 20 Lean back and twist 20 Bridge 100 Pullins Jog 30 mins	**Exercise** Abs 100 Reverse curls 20 Supermans 20 Lean back and twist 20 Bridge 100 Pullins Interval Training	
Gratitude diary	**Gratitude diary**	**Gratitude diary**	

bodyrescue

Week 7

Your Body Rescue
Weekly Plan

Weekly Plan diary

	Monday	Tuesday	Wednesday
Meditation	Visualise goals	Fears	Guilt
Exercise	Abs 100 Reverse curls 26 Supermans 26 Lean back and twist 20 Bridge 100 Pullins Bike ride 30 mins	Abs 100 Reverse curls 26 Supermans 26 Lean back and twist 20 Bridge 100 Pullins Resistance training	Abs 100 Reverse curls 26 Supermans 26 Lean back and twist 20 Bridge 100 Pullins Swim 30 mins
	Breakfast Psyllium husks, spirulina, aloe vera. Hot water and lemon. Fruit salad. **Snack** Yogurt, milled flaxseeds and agave nectar. **Lunch** Lasagne **Snack** Psyllium husks, spirulina, Nakd bar **Supper** Greek salad, glass of wine.	**Gratitude diary**	**Gratitude diary**
	Gratitude diary		

Meditation Goals every day **Gratitude diary**			
Exercise 3 cardio 30-45mins			
1 Interval training			
Yoga			
1 Resistance training			
100 Reverse curls			
26 Supermans			
26 Lean back and twist			
20 Bridge			
100 Pullins			
Eating As above plus 1 spirit or 1 small glass organic wine. (One for the week.)			

Thursday	Friday	Saturday	Sunday
Meditation Sabotage	**Meditation** Stress	**Meditation** Visualise goals	**Day off exercise**
Exercise Abs 100 Reverse curls 26 Supermans 26 Lean back and twist 20 Bridge 100 Pullins Yoga	**Exercise** Abs 100 Reverse curls 26 Supermans 26 Lean back and twist 20 Bridge 100 Pullins Jog 30 mins	**Exercise** Abs 100 Reverse curls 26 Supermans 26 Lean back and twist 20 Bridge 100 Pullins Interval training	
Gratitude diary	**Gratitude diary**	**Gratitude diary**	

bodyrescue

Week 8

Your Body Rescue Weekly Plan

	Monday	Tuesday	Wednesday
	Meditation Visualise goals	**Meditation** Fears	**Meditation** Guilt
	Exercise Abs Extended plank 30 seconds 50 Superman pull ins 10 Extended plank knee to opposite knee 50 Scissor sit up 10 Lean backs 50 Heel taps Bike ride 30 mins	**Exercise** Abs Extended plank 30 seconds 50 Superman pull ins 10 Extended plank knee to opposite knee 50 Scissor sit up 10 Lean backs 50 Heel taps Resistance training	**Exercise** Abs Extended plank 30 seconds 50 Superman pull ins 10 Extended plank knee to opposite knee 50 Scissor sit up 10 Lean backs 50 Heel taps Swim 30 mins
	Breakfast Psyllium husks, spirulina, aloe vera. Hot water and lemon. Fruit salad. **Snack** Yogurt, milled flaxseeds and agave nectar **Lunch** Prawn stir fry with noodles **Snack** Psyllium husks, spirulina, Nakd bar **Supper** Lentil shepherd's pie; glass of wine	**Gratitude diary**	**Gratitude diary**
	Gratitude diary		

Weekly Plan diary

Meditation Goals every day **Gratitude diary**			
Exercise 3 cardio 30-45mins			
1 Interval training			
1 Resistance training			
Extended plank 30 secs			
50 Superman pull ins			
10 Extended plank knee to opposite knee			
50 Scissor sit up			
10 Lean backs			
50 Heel taps			
Yoga			
Eating As above			

Thursday	Friday	Saturday	Sunday
Meditation	**Meditation**	**Meditation**	**Day off exercise**
Sabotage	Stress	Visualise goals	
Exercise	**Exercise**	**Exercise**	
Abs	Abs	Abs	
Extended plank 30 seconds	Extended plank 30 seconds	Extended plank 30 seconds	
50 Superman pull ins	50 Superman pull ins	50 Superman pull ins	
10 Extended plank knee to opposite knee	10 Extended plank knee to opposite knee	10 Extended plank knee to opposite knee	
50 Scissor sit up	50 Scissor sit up	50 Scissor sit up	
10 Lean backs	10 Lean backs	10 Lean backs	
50 Heel taps	50 Heel taps	50 Heel taps	
Yoga	Jog 30 mins	Interval training	
Gratitude diary	**Gratitude diary**	**Gratitude diary**	

bodyrescue

Week 9	Monday	Tuesday	Wednesday
Your Body Rescue Weekly Plan	**Meditation** Visualise goals	**Meditation** Fears	**Meditation** Guilt
	Exercise Abs 30 Reverse curls 10 Supermans 6 Lean back and twist 5 Bridge 50 Pullins	**Exercise** Abs 30 Reverse curls 10 Supermans 6 Lean back and twist 5 Bridge 50 Pullins Resistance training	**Exercise** Abs 30 Reverse curls 10 Supermans 6 Lean back and twist 5 Bridge 50 Pullins
	Breakfast Psyllium husks, spirulina, aloe vera. Hot water and lemon. Fruit salad. **Snack** Yogurt, milled flaxseeds and agave nectar. **Lunch** Salad Niçoise **Snack** Psyllium husks, spirulina, Nakd bar **Supper** Butternut squash risotto; vodka and orange	**Gratitude diary**	**Gratitude diary**
	Gratitude diary		

Weekly Plan diary

Meditation Goals every day **Gratitude diary**			
Exercise			
3 cardio workouts 30-45mins			
Yoga at home with meditation			
Extended plank 30 secs			
50 Superman pull ins			
10 Extended plank knee to opposite knee			
10 Lean backs			
50 Heel taps			
2 Resistance training a week			
Eating Same as week above			

Thursday	Friday	Saturday	Sunday
Meditation Sabotage	**Meditation** Stress	**Meditation** Visualise goals	**Day off exercise**
Exercise Abs Extended plank 40 seconds; 60 Superman pull ins 14 Extended plank knee to opposite knee 60 Scissor sit up 14 Lean backs 60 Heel taps Yoga	**Exercise** Abs Extended plank 40 seconds; 60 Superman pull ins 14 Extended plank knee to opposite knee 60 Scissor sit up 14 Lean backs 60 Heel taps Jog 30 mins	**Exercise** Abs Extended plank 40 seconds; 60 Superman pull ins 14 Extended plank knee to opposite knee 60 Scissor sit up 14 Lean backs 60 Heel taps Interval training	
Gratitude diary	**Gratitude diary**	**Gratitude diary**	

bodyrescue

Week 10

Your Body Rescue
Weekly Plan

(b·r)

	Monday	**Tuesday**	**Wednesday**
	Meditation Visualise goals	**Meditation** Fears	**Meditation** Guilt
	Exercise Abs Extended plank 50 seconds 70 Superman pull ins 16 Extended plank knee to opposite knee 70 Scissor sit up 16 Lean backs 70 Heel taps Bike ride 30 mins	**Exercise** Abs Extended plank 50 seconds 70 Superman pull ins 16 Extended plank knee to opposite knee 70 Scissor sit up 16 Lean backs 70 Heel taps Resistance training	**Exercise** Abs Extended plank 50 seconds 70 Superman pull ins 16 Extended plank knee to opposite knee 70 Scissor sit up 16 Lean backs 70 Heel taps Swim 30 mins
	Breakfast Psyllium husks, spirulina, aloe vera. Hot water and lemon. Apple, carrot and ginger juice. **Snack** Cashew nuts and raisins. **Lunch** Sweet potato with roasted veg. **Snack** Psyllium husks, spirulina, Nakdbar. **Supper** Sea bream and vegetables	**Gratitude diary**	**Gratitude diary**
	Gratitude diary		

Weekly Plan diary

Meditation Goals every day **Gratitude diary**			
Exercise 3 cardio 30-45mins			
2 Interval training			
2 Resistance training			
Abdominals every day			
Extended plank 50 secs			
70 Superman pull ins			
16 Extended plank knee to opposite knee			
70 Scissor sit up			
16 Lean backs			
70 Heel taps			
Eating Detox as week 1			

Thursday	Friday	Saturday	Sunday
Meditation Sabotage.	**Meditation** Stress.	**Meditation** Visualise goals	Day off exercise
Exercise Abs Extended plank 50 seconds 70 Superman pull ins 16 Extended plank knee to opposite knee 70 Scissor sit up 16 Lean backs 70 Heel taps Yoga **Gratitude diary**	**Exercise** Abs Extended plank 50 seconds 70 Superman pull ins 16 Extended plank knee to opposite knee 70 Scissor sit up 16 Lean backs 70 Heel taps Jog 30 mins **Gratitude diary**	**Exercise** Abs Extended plank 50 seconds 70 Superman pull ins 16 Extended plank knee to opposite knee 70 Scissor sit up 16 Lean backs 70 Heel taps Interval training **Gratitude diary**	

bodyrescue

Week 11

Your Body Rescue Weekly Plan

	Monday	Tuesday	Wednesday
Meditation	Visualise goals	Fears.	Guilt.
Exercise	Abs Extended plank 60 seconds 80 Superman pull ins 18 Extended plank knee to opposite knee 80 Scissor sit up 18 Lean backs 80 Heel taps Bike ride 30 mins	Abs Extended plank 60 seconds 80 Superman pull ins 18 Extended plank knee to opposite knee 80 Scissor sit up 18 Lean backs 80 Heel taps Resistance training	Abs Extended plank 60 seconds 80 Superman pull ins 18 Extended plank knee to opposite knee 80 Scissor sit up 18 Lean backs 80 Heel taps Swim 30 mins
	Breakfast Psyllium husks, spirulina, aloe vera. Hot water and lemon. Yogurt and bananas. **Snack** cashew nuts and raisins **Lunch** Rice salad. **Snack** Psyllium husks, spirulina, Nakd bar. **Supper** Salmon and vegetables	**Gratitude diary**	**Gratitude diary**
	Gratitude diary		

Weekly Plan diary

Meditation Goals every day **Gratitude diary**			
Exercise 3 cardio workouts a week - 30-45mins			
2 Resistance training			
2 Interval training			
Extended plank 60 secs			
80 Superman pull ins			
18 Extended plank knee to opposite knee			
80 Scissor sit up			
18 Lean backs			
80 Heel taps			
Yoga			
Eating Detox as week 2			

Thursday	Friday	Saturday	Sunday
Meditation Sabotage.	**Meditation** Stress.	**Meditation** Visualise goals	**Day off exercise**
Exercise Abs Extended plank 60 seconds 80 Superman pull ins 18 Extended plank knee to opposite knee 80 Scissor sit up 18 Lean backs 80 Heel taps Yoga	**Exercise** Abs Extended plank 60 seconds 80 Superman pull ins 18 Extended plank knee to opposite knee 80 Scissor sit up 18 Lean backs 80 Heel taps Jog 30 mins	**Exercise** Abs Extended plank 60 seconds 80 Superman pull ins 18 Extended plank knee to opposite knee 80 Scissor sit up 18 Lean backs 80 Heel taps Interval training	
Gratitude diary	**Gratitude diary**	**Gratitude diary**	

bodyrescue

Week 12 | Monday | Tuesday | Wednesday

Week 12	Monday	Tuesday	Wednesday
Meditation	Visualise goals	Fears	Guilt
Exercise	Abs Extended plank 70 seconds 80 Superman pull ins 120 Extended plank knee to opposite knee 90 Scissor sit up 20 Lean backs 80 Heel taps Plank 90 seconds Bike ride 30 mins	Abs Extended plank 70 seconds 80 Superman pull ins 120 Extended plank knee to opposite knee 90 Scissor sit up 20 Lean backs 80 Heel taps Plank 90 seconds Resistance training	Abs Extended plank 70 seconds 80 Superman pull ins 120 Extended plank knee to opposite knee 90 Scissor sit up 20 Lean backs 80 Heel taps Plank 90 seconds Swim 30 mins
Breakfast	Psyllium husks, spirulina, aloe vera. Hot water and lemon. Yogurt and bananas.		
Snack	Cashew nuts and raisins.		
Lunch	Rice salad		
Snack	Psyllium husks, spirulina, Nakd bar		
Supper	Salmon and vegetables		
	Gratitude diary	**Gratitude diary**	**Gratitude diary**

Your Body Rescue Weekly Plan

Weekly Plan diary

Meditation
Goals every day
Gratitude diary

Exercise			
3 cardio 30-45mins			
2 Interval training			
2 Resistance training			
Abs			
Extended Plank 70 secs			
80 Superman Pull ins			
120 Extended plank knee to opposite knee			
90 Scissor sit up			
20 Lean backs			
80 Heel taps			
1 Yoga			

Eating
Same as week 5

Thursday	Friday	Saturday	Sunday
Meditation Sabotage	**Meditation** Stress	**Meditation** Visualise goals	**Day off exercise**
Exercise Abs Extended plank 70 seconds 80 Superman pull ins 120 Extended plank knee to opposite knee 90 Scissor sit up 20 Lean backs 80 Heel taps Yoga	**Exercise** Abs Extended plank 70 seconds 80 Superman pull ins 120 Extended plank knee to opposite knee 90 Scissor sit up 20 Lean backs 80 Heel taps Jog 30 mins	**Exercise** Abs Extended plank 70 seconds 80 Superman pull ins 120 Extended plank knee to opposite knee 90 Scissor sit up 20 Lean backs 80 Heel taps Interval training	
Gratitude diary	**Gratitude diary**	**Gratitude diary**	

bodyrescue

Maintenance programme

Week 13	Monday	Tuesday	Wednesday
Your Body Rescue Weekly Plan	**Meditation** Relaxation	**Meditation** Relaxation	**Meditation** Relaxation
	Exercise Abs Extended plank 70 seconds 80 Superman pull ins 120 Extended plank knee to opposite knee 90 Scissor sit up 20 Lean backs 80 Heel taps Bike ride 30 mins	**Exercise** Abs Extended plank 70 seconds 80 Superman pull ins 120 Extended plank knee to opposite knee 90 Scissor sit up 20 Lean backs 80 Heel taps Resistance training	**Exercise** Abs Extended plank 70 seconds 80 Superman pull ins 120 Extended plank knee to opposite knee 90 Scissor sit up 20 Lean backs 80 Heel taps Swim 30 mins
	Breakfast Psyllium husks, spirulina, aloe vera. Hot water and lemon. Yogurt and bananas **Snack** cashew nuts and raisins **Lunch** Rice salad. **Snack** Psyllium husks, spirulina, Nakd bar **Supper** Salmon and vegetables	**Gratitude diary**	**Gratitude diary**
	Gratitude diary		

Weekly Plan diary

Meditation Relaxation **Gratitude diary**			
Exercise 3 cardio 30-45mins			
2 Interval training			
2 resistance training			
Abs			
Extended plank 70 secs			
80 Superman pull ins			
120 Extended plank knee to opposite knee			
90 Scissor sit up			
20 Lean backs			
80 Heel taps			
1 Yoga			
Eating Same as week 6 plus 1 cheat day a week - anything you like			

Thursday	Friday	Saturday	Sunday
Meditation Relaxation	**Meditation** Relaxation	**Meditation** Relaxation	**Day off exercise**
Exercise Abs Extended plank 70 seconds 80 Superman pull ins 120 Extended plank knee to opposite knee 90 Scissor sit up 20 Lean backs 80 Heel taps Yoga	**Exercise** Abs Extended plank 70 seconds 80 Superman pull ins 120 Extended plank knee to opposite knee 90 Scissor sit up 20 Lean backs 80 Heel taps Jog 30 mins	**Exercise** Abs Extended plank 70 seconds 80 Superman pull ins 120 Extended plank knee to opposite knee 90 Scissor sit up 20 Lean backs 80 Heel taps Interval training	**Cheat day** Have any meal you like but if you still feel addicted to certain foods i.e.: once you eat them you can't stop, go a few weeks longer until you have control. It may be certain foods won't ever agree with you, but there are always yummy alternatives.
Gratitude diary	**Gratitude diary**	**Gratitude diary**	

bodyrescue

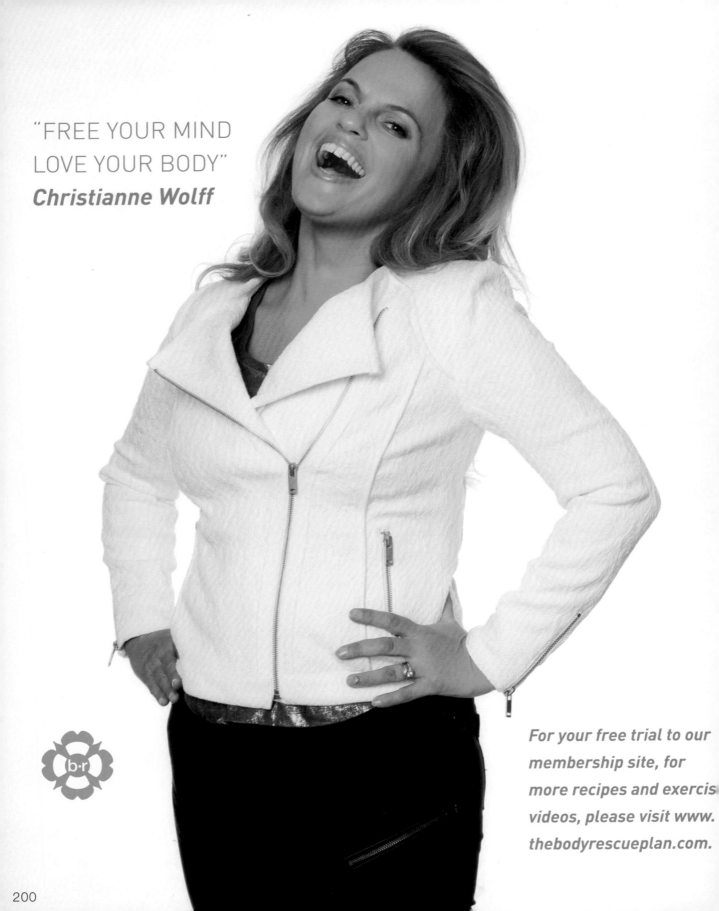

"FREE YOUR MIND
LOVE YOUR BODY"
Christianne Wolff

For your free trial to our membership site, for more recipes and exercis videos, please visit www. thebodyrescueplan.com.